The
Healing
Power
of
Faith

*Science Explores
Medicine's Last
Great Frontier*

Harold G. Koenig, M.D.

With Additional Research by Carol
and Malcolm McConnell

Simon & Schuster

SIMON & SCHUSTER
Rockefeller Center
1230 Avenue of the Americas
New York, NY 10020

DESIGNED BY DEIRDRE C. AMTHOR

Manufactured in the United States of America

10 9 8 7 6 5 4 3 2 1

Library of Congress Cataloging-in-Publication Data
Koenig, Harold George.
    The healing power of faith : science explores medicine's
last great frontier / Harold G. Koenig ; with additional research
by Carol and Malcolm McConnell.
        p.   cm.
    Includes bibliographical references and index.
    1. Health—Religious aspects.   I. Title.
BL65.M4K63   1999
291.1'78321—dc21   98-32079
                                              CIP

ISBN 0-684-85296-9

※

Acknowledgments

I wish to express my sincere appreciation to all the people who generously shared their personal stories in this book.

I greatly appreciate and owe a debt of gratitude to my colleagues at the Duke University Center for the Study of Religion/Spirituality and Health, especially Linda George, Ph.D., Harvey Cohen, M.D., and David Larson, M.D., who have worked with me during the years of research that underlie this book.

I also wish to thank the staff of the John Templeton Foundation, particularly John M. Templeton, Jr., M.D., and Charles L. Harper, Jr., D. Phil., who also have been staunch supporters of my work. Carol McConnell wishes to thank the John Templeton Foundation for the research grant she received.

I also want to thank Simon & Schuster senior editor Roslyn Siegel, for her insightful guidance, and my agent, Kristen Wainwright, for her hard work.

Finally, I would like to thank Charmin, my beautiful wife, who has had to endure my passionate love for my work that has often taken me away from home and my two precious children, Jordan (age ten) and Rebekah (age four). They have truly bolstered me through my own tough times and freed me to pursue my dreams.

To Sir John Templeton

✳ Contents

10 Contents

*

Chapter One

✳

Science, Religion, and Health

In February 1996, I chaired a symposium on "Social and Religious Factors Affecting Health" at the annual meeting of the American Association for the Advancement of Science. A professor from a prestigious university approached me during a coffee break at the Baltimore conference room.

"Doctor Koenig, how did someone with your background ever become interested in religion?" he asked.

"That's a tough question," I replied.

After all, I'm a physician who has spent years mastering several complex specialties. The Association is widely viewed as the world's most prominent science organization. And natural science, with its immutable laws and formulae, is the foundation of modern medicine, while religion, by definition, deals with inexplicable *super*natural powers and events. He no doubt wondered what had made me diverge from my grounding in biomedical science to venture into the intangible realm of religious faith.

A Voyage of Discovery

My career has been more a voyage of discovery than a predictable linear progression from student to clinician to medical professor and researcher. During this twenty-year odyssey, I've worked as a hospital orderly and registered nurse, often in intimate contact with sick people. I have been certified in family medicine, psychiatry, geriatric medicine, and geriatric psychiatry. My clinical practice has brought me newborn babies and their mothers as well as elderly people in their final weeks, and the full range of physical and emotional illness between infancy and old age. I've encountered people whose bodies were ravaged by disease, but who somehow remained optimistic and emotionally healthy, and others who were so wounded by stress and emotional trauma that the ensuing depression destroyed their lives.

Today I am director of Duke University's Center for the Study of Religion/Spirituality and Health, the world's first major research facility to comprehensively study the impact of people's religious life on their physical and emotional health.

Struggling to answer my colleague's question that February afternoon in Baltimore, I recognized an important aspect of my professional life: It was my patients who led me to explore the previously underinvestigated connection between health and religious faith. Without question, I have learned more about the resilience of the human spirit in the face of crushing adversity from the people I treated than I ever did from textbooks or medical school lectures.

An Unusual Alcoholic: Lee's Story

I met the first of these patients—a middle-aged man named Lee Daugherty—in November 1981, when I was a third-year medical student at the University of California at San Francisco. As part of my Internal Medicine rotation, I covered rounds at San Francisco General Hospital. Lee had been admitted on Halloween, suffering from severe complications of alcoholism.

"Good morning, Mr. Daugherty," I said to the gaunt man hunched beneath the sheets. His hair was long, his face haggard. Lee's chart reported he had been living on the streets of the Mission district for years. His daily alcohol consumption was estimated at more than six pints of cheap fortified wine. The night before, he had suffered a seizure, tumbled headlong into the street, and sprawled there in the cold drizzle, unable to rise. Lee's diagnosis included cirrhosis, neurological involvement, and complications of malnutrition. His blackouts and seizures were the most alarming symptoms, a probable indication of brain damage.*

Lee rolled over and stared at me with red-rimmed eyes. "What time is it?" he grumbled.

"Just after seven." Rounds on this ward started early.

"Can I have some coffee?" he asked as I felt his rapid, uneven pulse.

Before rounds that morning, my instructors had described Lee as a typical "terminal" alcoholic. My initial examination seemed to confirm that grim prognosis. But, unlike some of my fellow students, and because I'd worked wards as an orderly and nurse, I saw my patients as real people, not just interesting cases. With Lee, I was gripped by the need to help someone who was suffering, but also by a sense of futility. I knew that Lee's level of alcoholism could rarely be cured. People like Lee are not "problem drinkers," but so profoundly addicted that they suffer life-threatening convulsions if deprived of alcohol. Almost inevitably, the disease crushes their spirits until they're sluggishly fatalistic. But I saw a lively spark in Lee's blue eyes. I fetched him a cup of coffee.

Lee sat up in bed and examined me with new interest. "Doctors never did that before," he said, cuddling his coffee cup.

"You've had a terrible time, Lee," I said, consulting his chart, "and you're very sick. I'm recommending we keep you here as long as possible. You just can't go straight back to the street."

"I'll be okay once my legs get better, Doc," he said.

Even though I was as overworked as any medical student, I stayed with him a while longer. "You will *not* be okay, Lee," I said, placing my hand on his thin arm. "If you start drinking again, you'll be dead before summer."

Lee savored the last of his coffee. "I'll be all right," he insisted. "God has a purpose in my life."

*I have rendered meetings with patients and other personal stories in a narrative form with the permission of those involved. When noted, I have changed people's names to protect their privacy.

His confident words surprised me. Lee Daugherty was one of the "lost souls" who can be found on inner-city streets across the country. Yet he seemed to firmly believe that God would intervene in his life. "How can you be so sure?" I was preoccupied with hard medical science, not the mysteries of faith.

"God has a plan for me," Lee repeated. "Last night, layin' there in the gutter, I saw kids in Halloween costumes going up Mission, and I thought about my life. . . ."

Lee had been born in rural Oklahoma in 1931, at the peak of the Dust Bowl drought that sent thousands of Okie immigrants to California. His father had died when Lee was an infant, and his mother soon fell ill. He and his brother were raised in foster homes. By his twenties, Lee was one of the country's millions of functional alcoholics, working as a cook, successfully hiding his growing addiction. Alcohol, however, eventually overpowered his life, and by his forties Lee was living on the desolate streets of San Francisco's Mission district, panhandling for rotgut wine. He didn't drink for pleasure anymore, but just to "keep from getting sick."

Lying against the cold curb, his legs paralyzed, Lee had prayed for guidance. "Lord, if this is all there is to life," he had moaned, speaking directly to God, "I just want it to end. But if there is more, can you show me?"

He had virtually hit rock bottom the night before in that gutter. Yet now he seemed serene. "I think the Lord is showing me the way out of this mess," he said confidently.

"Maybe so," I agreed to keep his mood up. "But you're still going to need a place to stay when they discharge you. And you're going to have to go through detox again."

Lee nodded. "This time I'm going to make it, Doc."

You can appreciate my skepticism. Lee Daugherty had already been through half a dozen detoxification programs. He'd also tried Alcoholics Anonymous. He'd always gone back to drinking. Yet somehow he was convinced that the Lord would lift the burden of his disease. I suddenly recalled a passage from Sigmund Freud that had impressed me as a premed student. Religion, Freud had proclaimed, was the "univer-

*

sal obsessional neurosis of humanity." This undoubtedly hopeless alcoholic seemed gripped by just the type of delusion Freud had identified. *Well, I thought, at least Lee's faith brings him some comfort.*

I managed to keep him in the hospital for almost a week so that his withdrawal symptoms could be tempered by medication. And I helped find him a hotel room near the detox center. I also gave Lee my phone number and asked him to stay in touch, secretly fearful that I'd receive a call from a cop who'd found the number on Lee's lifeless body on the street.

Imagine my surprise when Lee called me that spring. "I'm getting married, Doc," he announced proudly. Lee had met Charlotte in the San Francisco General detox program. Like him, she had an abiding faith that God would free her of alcohol dependence. Together they were struggling through each day, determined to let their faith guide them to the inner healing necessary to break the grip of alcoholism. When I left California to begin my family medicine residency at the University of Missouri in Columbia, Lee and Charlotte Daugherty were sober and working, saving their money in hopes of buying a home.

"Congratulations," I told Lee.

"We couldn't have done it without God's help," Lee said, noting that they began and ended each day reading scripture. "I really like Ecclesiastes," he added. " 'To every thing there is a season . . . a time to weep and a time to laugh. . . .' This is our time to get well."

Proud of my new M.D., with boundless confidence in the power of medical science, I attributed Lee's remission more to the techniques and medications of the detox counselors than to the healing power of his faith. But his experience had also sparked an ember of curiosity. Would he and Charlotte have managed to salvage their lives if they hadn't possessed such a deep faith?

A Lesson in Optimism: Ruby and Bill's Story

Ruby and Bill Clevenger were also patients who sharpened my interest in the health benefits of religious faith. During my family medicine residency in Missouri in the early 1980s, I often visited patients in their homes. The Clevengers lived in an old frame farmhouse in Callaway County. Bill Clevenger was eighty-one when we met. He had the strong, gnarled hands and weathered face of a man who'd worked hard his whole life, but he was now incapacitated by emphysema, and also suffered increasing deafness. Ruby, then near seventy, had a glow to her cheeks and a serenely cheerful manner.

Despite Bill's health problems, they welcomed me to their home with the genuine graciousness that comes naturally to many country people. As we sat in the small parlor, I discreetly studied them both for any signs of melancholy that might indicate an underlying depression.

Doctors learn early in their careers that serious, sometimes crippling depression afflicts many elderly people suffering from chronic physical illness. Although about 5 percent of the general population suffers from depression, almost *half* of those people with severe health problems become depressed. Many sick older people abandon hope that their lives will ever get better. Nervous and irritable, they lose interest in activities they once enjoyed, often have difficulty concentrating, withdraw from others, and feel worthless. Indeed, the severe depression that frequently follows physical illness can delay healing and provoke premature death.

With his emphysema growing worse and threatening to make him housebound, and his deafness deepening his isolation, Bill Clevenger was a likely candidate for depression. But the handsome elderly man sitting across the parlor on the chintz-covered easy chair was obviously alert, beaming with friendly interest in my visit.

"Finally getting some nice spring weather," I commented.

Bill cupped his ear and leaned toward Ruby. "Ask him to please speak so that I can hear him," he said in a loud, toneless voice.

"Sorry," I said, speaking louder. I was prepared for Bill to slip into a sour lament about his failing health.

But he grinned warmly. "I like to talk if I can hear what people say." He explained that his hearing had deteriorated over many years, beginning when he was a youngster working with explosives on the railroad. "But I can still sing my hymns at church," Bill added.

"We're Baptists," Ruby interjected, "but we've gone to all kinds of different churches over the years."

There were religious pictures on the walls and end tables. They were standard, inexpensive pastel-tone prints—The Last Supper, Jesus alone in prayer, the Virgin and Baby Jesus. "I get them at rummage sales," Ruby said. "They always make me feel good."

The Clevengers seemed to take comfort in religion and church worship. But I had no way to gauge the impact of this faith on their physical health and outlook. However, it was clear that neither one suffered from depression. Bill's laugh was hardy and unfeigned; Ruby's plans for their summer vegetable garden rang with cheerful optimism. But it was when they brought out their photo album that I discovered just how well Bill and Ruby had coped with an often difficult life.

"We've been foster parents for years," Ruby said, opening the album to reveal snapshots of the Clevengers and a remarkable number of children on picnics or grouped around a Christmas tree. Some of the children had crutches; several were of mixed race.

"We took the kids other people didn't want," Bill said.

"They're all precious in the eyes of the Lord," Ruby added, fondly turning the pages to linger on the dozens of young faces that had passed through their lives. She showed me the six teenage girls they had cared for at the same time several years earlier. Some of them had been abused. All had come from shattered families.

Bill Clevenger beamed, studying the girls' pictures. "We didn't always have a lot to give them except a warm house, clean clothes, and good hot food," he said.

"And love," Ruby added. "They all got plenty of that."

I was surprised that the Clevengers were still active foster parents, despite Bill's condition, which demanded a lot of care from Ruby. Leafing through the album, I realized that both Bill and Ruby Clevenger enjoyed a healthy self-respect, yet were completely free of the self-absorption that grips many elderly people with health problems.

We were still looking at the pictures when the kitchen door opened and a slight, dark-haired girl of about ten entered, moving tentatively in the presence of a stranger.

"Cindy," Ruby said, taking the child's hand. "Say your hello to Dr. Koenig."

"Cindy's our daughter," Bill said proudly.

Cindy was mentally retarded. Ruby gently explained that they had adopted the girl after she had spent her first three years in their home as a foster child and it became obvious her disability would make adoption elsewhere very difficult.

"She's God's child," Ruby said with surprising conviction, taking Cindy onto her lap.

How many old people with their problems would have happily assumed such a responsibility?

Over the coming months, I often visited the Clevengers. Bill's physical condition did not improve. But both he and Ruby retained their uncomplaining cheerfulness. And they always made some reference to the role of religion in their lives.

Somehow, I realized, their faith is shielding them from depression.

Soothing Fears: Ruth's Story

As my residency continued, I became convinced that there were many people like the Daughertys and the Clevengers who used religious faith to cope with otherwise crushing problems.

I'll never forget Mrs. Edna Hanson (name changed), whom I met in the university hospital the day before she had surgery. Mrs. Hanson, a widow of seventy-five, was a ten-year breast cancer survivor who had later received a hip replacement. As sometimes happens, the artificial hip joint did not graft well. Now she faced the same painful surgery again.

That afternoon I found her sitting in a chair at the window of her hospital room, quietly reading the Bible.

"I hope I'm not intruding," I said.

She slid her bookmark into place and smiled. "You're not disturbing me at all," she said. "I was just reading Matthew and Luke."

After we discussed her physical therapy schedule, I became curious about her religious faith. Unlike other patients I'd encountered confronting major surgery with a questionable prognosis, she showed no obvious anxiety.

"How do you feel about tomorrow?" I asked. "It must be hard going through all this again."

She thought a moment. "Well, I got real angry when they said I'd have to come back for a new operation," she said with some embarrassment. "Then I got real sad, just sort of blue for a week or so. I lost my appetite and I cried at night when I couldn't sleep." She reached for her Bible. "Then I began reading my scripture. I like to say the Lord's Prayer out loud, just the way Jesus taught it to the disciples. It's calmed me down completely."

"You certainly look calm," I agreed.

"The Bible just brings me comfort," she said.

Indeed, her pulse rate and blood pressure were normal. Mrs. Hanson's case history stated that her husband of forty-six years had died three years earlier and her two grown children, who lived out of state, were unable to be with her. She was emotionally isolated as she faced the uncertainty of this new operation, yet coped with the stress amazingly well.

As I left the room, she switched on the table lamp and took up her Bible. The image of that elderly woman sitting alone with her scriptures remained with me on my rounds. Pre-op patients often required medication to calm them, but not Mrs. Hanson. Was she a rare case, or did her faith bring her both emotional and physical peace? Were Lee and Charlotte Daugherty and the Clevengers also exceptional?

What Medical School Didn't Teach Me

Nothing I'd been taught in four years of medical school or the first two years of my residency even hinted that religious faith could break the grip of addiction, shield people from depression, or calm them at times of emotional trauma. In fact, there were many examples in the medical literature that echoed Freud by implying religion was a neurotic crutch of little practical use at times of severe stress. In a 1960 report entitled "The Meaning of Religion to Older People," geriatric expert Dr. Nila

Kirkpatrick Covalt had found no evidence to support the accepted belief that "people turn to religion as they grow older." As to the benefits
of scriptural reading for the hospitalized patient, Covalt was almost
scornful: "We physicians have learned that when a patient brings a
Bible with him to the hospital and keeps it displayed, this action is a
sign of anticipated trouble from an insecure individual."[1]

Covalt described ignorant patients from "fringe" religious sects who
brandished their Bibles and became so uncooperative that they upset
hospital routine.

But the religious patients I had encountered certainly did not fit this
pattern. Faith seemed to have brought the Daughertys, the Clevengers,
and Mrs. Hanson a degree of protection from physical and emotional
illness. I began to wonder if modern medicine, in its quest to shine the
light of scientific truth on the last vestiges of medicine-show quackery,
was ignoring the potential healing power of religious faith?

Although I became intrigued by this question, I recognized that my
experience with religious patients had been limited to what we call
"anecdotal" observation. But I also knew that every breakthrough in
medicine had begun with such random observations that led to hypotheses, which eventually stood up to the stringent testing of the scientific method. Edward Jenner observed that dairymaids were immune
to smallpox because they contracted the less virulent cowpox; this led
to the discovery of "vaccination" (which derives from the Latin word
for cow). Sir Alexander Fleming noticed that common bread mold,
penicillium notatum, killed bacteria in a petri dish; that chance observation sparked the development of antibiotics, which have revolutionized
medicine. But how could I test the hypothesis that religious faith had
inherent healing power?

Scientific research demands rigorous investigative methods and ex-
acting, neutral peer review of findings and conclusions, which other researchers can then replicate. Launching such a disciplined research
study into the health benefits of religious faith in the mid-1980s was
scary. I was a young resident and sure didn't want to get branded as an
"unscientific" religious zealot.

*

Applying Science to Religious Faith

So I began my research career with a small investigation. Geriatric and psychiatric studies had established that fear of death could cause chronic stress that diminished the quality of life of older people. Yet among my religious patients facing life-threatening illness, I'd noticed many whose faith shielded them from this morbid preoccupation. Therefore I decided to investigate the relationship between religious belief and practice and death anxiety among several hundred elderly people attending senior lunch programs.[2]

To test my hypothesis that religious faith and practices such as prayer, scriptural reading, and church attendance might help older people cope with several forms of stress, including death anxiety, I circulated a twenty-six-item questionnaire among the subjects. I was trying to assess their religious belief and activities, their feelings about death, their tolerance of stress and what social scientists call general "coping."

To probe their reliance on faith under stress, I asked, "When you are facing a difficult situation, how likely are you to use prayer to help you deal with the situation?" They could respond with "unlikely," "somewhat likely," and "very likely." I also instructed them, "Think of the most stressful experience you had in recent months. To what extent did you use your religious beliefs in coping with this stressful experience?" The possible responses ranged from "very little" to "very much."

In addition, I asked about their level of community activity and their involvement in their church congregation or faith community. I wanted to separate nonreligious activity such as club membership from purely religious practices such as participation in worship service.

To measure their level of death anxiety, I asked: "There are many feelings people have about death. How do you feel?" People could respond on a scale ranging from "fearful and anxious" to "no fear or anxiety."

I assessed the subjects' physical health, because research showed that people suffering serious illness are often fearful of death. Responses ranged from "sick and disabled" to "very healthy, not disabled."

After posting all the responses and checking their validity with recognized statistical procedures, I was surprised and heartened by the findings. Those elderly people who were "very likely" to rely on religious faith and prayer when under stress were much more likely to report little or no fear about death, when compared with their peers for whom faith and prayer were less important.

This difference was statistically significant: 10.3 percent of the deeply religious people experienced death anxiety compared with almost 25 percent of the less religious. People who were actively involved in their religious communities also reported less fear of death. But my findings suggested that it was personal faith and not necessarily religious activity that helped these older people deal with stressful problems and allowed them to cope with fears of death. Religious faith was especially important among the chronically ill and disabled older people.

The Center for the Study of Religion/Spirituality and Health

Looking back, that first research project was indeed modest. However, I was encouraged that my findings were both statistically significant and had passed the rigor of the peer review process. In the mid-1980s, the connection between health and spirituality, and research on other "mind-body" relationships, had not yet achieved widespread acceptance.

Many of my colleagues tried to steer me away from what they saw as a marginal field of investigation. To them, the only demonstrable links between faith and health were the dubious practices of greedy television faith healers. I understood their concern. During my training in geriatric medicine, psychiatry, and geriatric psychiatry in the 1980s, I was flooded by discoveries on the frontiers of molecular biology and brain chemistry. Medicine could now chart the progress of cancers and cardiovascular disease from the cellular level and devise bold new treatments for these dread illnesses. CT scans and MRI technology opened exquisite windows into the living body. Whole new classes of psychoactive medications had burst on the scene, allowing us to treat previously intractable conditions such as schizophrenia and bipolar disorder. I was in the middle of a new renaissance in scientific medicine.

But I continued to meet patients like the Daughertys and the Clevengers whose health had been clearly bolstered by their religious faith. Explaining this phenomenon in scientific terms has become my life's work. Since my first tentative faith-health research, I have led or participated in scores of much larger and more thorough studies. Eighteen years have passed since I met Lee Daugherty. As head of Duke University's Center for the Study of Religion/Spirituality and Health, I've seen research on religion and health evolve from pioneering studies by Duke faculty in the 1960s. Over the years, our center's scientists have led over fifty major research projects on the relationship between faith and health. More than seventy data-based, peer-reviewed papers published in medical and scientific journals have resulted from these projects.

Duke's center divides the role of religion/spirituality in health into three categories: "Illness Prevention," "Illness Recovery," and "Treatment/Health Services Use." Other research facilities, including the Mind-Body Medical Institute of the Harvard Medical School and Boston's Deaconess Hospital, have investigated the physiological effects of spiritual practices such as meditation. But our center has focused on the impact of traditional religious faith and practice—including individual prayer and congregational worship among American Christians and Jews—on physical health and emotional well-being.

These investigations have rigorously followed the established techniques of medical and social scientific research. My colleagues and I have avoided the delicate issue of the supernatural. For example, we don't try to establish the validity of faith healing, but we do investigate the therapeutic or healing power of people's religious faith. We certainly do not try to prove which religious or spiritual beliefs are more valid or correct in an absolute sense. Despite our differing individual faiths, we are scientists concerned with concrete data, not evangelists dealing with theological matters.

Many of the Duke Center's studies have produced groundbreaking findings:

- People who regularly attend church, pray individually, and read the Bible have significantly lower diastolic blood pressure than the less religious. Those with the lowest blood pressure both attend church and pray or study the Bible often.
- People who attend church regularly are hospitalized much less often than people who never or rarely participate in religious services.
- People with strong religious faith are less likely to suffer depression from stressful life events, and if they do, they are more likely to recover from depression than those who are less religious.
- The deeper a person's religious faith, the less likely he or she is to be crippled by depression during and after hospitalization for physical illness.
- Religious people have healthier lifestyles. They tend to avoid alcohol and drug abuse, risky sexual behavior, and other unhealthy habits.
- Elderly people with a deep, personal ("intrinsic") religious faith have a stronger sense of well-being and life satisfaction than their less religious peers. This may be due in part to the stable marriages and strong families religious people tend to build.
- People with strong faith who suffer from physical illness have significantly better health outcomes than less religious people.
- People who attend religious services regularly have stronger immune systems than their less religious counterparts. We found that people who went to church regularly had significantly lower blood levels of interleukin-6 (IL-6), which rises with unrelieved chronic stress. High levels of IL-6 reflect a weakened immune system, which, in turn, increases the risk of infection, autoimmune disease, and certain cancers.
- Religious people live longer. A growing body of research shows that religious people are both physically healthier into later life and live longer than their nonreligious counterparts. Religious faith appears to protect the elderly from the two major afflictions of later life, cardiovascular disease and cancer. In this regard, religion may be as significant a protective factor as not smoking in terms of survival and longevity.

Hundreds of major studies by other researchers have produced similar findings. For example, religious hip-fracture patients recover faster than their nonreligious counterparts. Older people who attend religious services avoid disability significantly longer than their nonattending peers. After open-heart surgery, patients who find comfort in their religious faith are three times more likely to survive than nonreligious patients. The risk of dying from all causes is up to 35 percent lower for people who attend religious services once or more a week than for those who attend less frequently.

Applying What We've Learned

What does all this research mean to you and your family? Probably more than you realize: The chances are you are already religious; the great majority of Americans are. Polls indicate that 96 percent of people believe in God or a universal spirit and that 90 percent pray.[3]

Some social scientists and journalists are convinced religion is enjoying a rebirth in America as Baby Boomers age and confront their own mortality. For example, Deborah Howell, Washington bureau chief of Newhouse News Service, recently noted in a C-SPAN television discussion: "The news media are finally getting it. Religion is the most important aspect of most people's lives." Certainly the runaway popularity of television shows such as *Touched by an Angel* and *Promised Land* indicate that millions of Americans are interested in spiritual matters.

But fewer than half of all Americans (43 percent) regularly attend religious services, even though research reveals that people who combine a strong personal faith with religious activity, including participation in worship service, receive the most significant health benefits of faith. The results of our research suggest it would be beneficial to increase your religious practices if this is compatible with your personal faith. Even if you lack strong faith, you might gain considerable health benefits by observing devoutly religious people and adopting some of their practices, perhaps community volunteer work. Later in the book, we will discuss the practical application of our research, even for those who lack religious belief entirely.

You will *not* find any pastoral advice or specific spiritual guidance in this book. Instead, I hope the personal stories I have shaped from case histories and linked to relevant research findings will allow you to reach conclusions about the contribution that faith and religious practice can make to your own health, healing, and well-being.

I want to emphasize that the concept of "Healing" used in the title of this book is not limited to the cure of physical disease or recovery from injury. When people suffer prolonged illness or disability, they often become slaves to the disease, which can dominate every aspect of their lives. I've met patients who surrender to illness and experience anguished desperation that far exceeds their physical pain. In some cases, we recognize this hopelessness as depression, which can further erode physical health and make recovery very difficult.

But others, like Bill Clevenger and Mrs. Hanson, use faith to place their physical conditions in perspective and give them the confidence needed to fight the illness.

We physicians do not fully understand the relationship between mind, body, and that intangible element known as spirit. But we treat religious people every day whose indomitable spirits and faith prevent their physical sickness from ruling their lives.

The nature of "Faith" mentioned in the title is described by many of my patients as the confident belief in a supreme being, which most call God. For them, God is loving and accessible. This is a God who listens to prayer, who responds, who desires good for humanity. This is an *intentional* God who sets goals we can strive toward to reach our highest potential in terms of physical, mental, and spiritual health—which aren't always achieved in that order. Those with faith in this God rarely feel lost or abandoned or experience the psychological anguish we call "anomie," a condition that afflicts millions in our fast-paced, affluent world.

What is the connection between the concepts of "Faith" and "Power" in the title?

People have told me that their faith gives them a tangible sense of mastery in their lives. When the inevitable stress of daily problems—illness, financial worries, personal conflicts—threatens to overwhelm religious people, they draw on a reserve of energy and motivation that allows them to persevere. They trust in God to fill the gap between what they could normally endure and what is actually required of them. They do not struggle alone, but rather see God as their active partner in the continuous struggle to achieve peace and balance in their lives.

Is this confidence in "the Healing Power of Faith" rational from a purely scientific perspective?

I recognize that research can neither prove nor disprove the reality of answered prayers or divine intercession. By definition, a supernatural event is beyond the reach of scientific investigation. And I also accept that my role as a physician and medical researcher is different from the clergy's. But, although scientists cannot demonstrate whether God exists and intervenes in people's lives, I have learned that we can certainly explore and chart in a scientific manner the *effect* of religious faith and practice on physical and emotional health.

Chapter Two

✳

Faith and Life Satisfaction

As a scientist, I've been impressed by the growing body of research evidence suggesting that deeply religious people are significantly happier about their lives than people who don't share as strong a faith. And as a specialist in geriatric medicine and in psychiatry, these findings hearten me.

Treating patients over the years, I've seen many people's later lives blighted by chronic anxiety and rancor, a bitter, ongoing disappointment. They feel isolated and useless; the decades spent at work and raising their families now seem bleak futility. The chronic emotional pain and stress of this dissatisfaction can trigger clinical depression, which in turn can worsen physical illness. If you visit a typical community nursing home, you'll find some of the residents openly despondent and glum, devoid of that precious quality psychologists call "life satisfaction" or emotional well-being.

But a large proportion of elderly people, either living in their own homes or in care facilities, are cheerful, optimistic, and seem to radiate inner peace and satisfaction with their lives. It's been my experience—confirmed in recent research studies—that these emotionally tranquil older people often possess a strong religious faith, which they practice through regular prayer and congregational worship. They seem to derive their personal satisfaction from the unshakable certainty that God has guided the events of their lives, both good and bad, and continues to do so in their later years.[1]

Living in a Benevolent Universe

I noted earlier that medical educators have often taught that religion is an irrelevant or even detrimental factor in physical and emotional well-being. But a growing body of research has established that religious people, both young and old, often enjoy the psychological and physical benefits of a positive emotional outlook. In the wake of research documenting the physical and emotional benefits of religious faith, the John Templeton Foundation began in 1995 to award American medical schools grants to develop courses on faith and medicine such as that developed by Thomas Corson, M.D., an internist and pediatrician at Johns Hopkins. The impressive data on the health benefits of faith have spurred a growing interest in the subject among medical students.[2]

I certainly don't mean to imply that religious people never worry or experience depression. But research has consistently shown they have the ability to rebound from negative mental states faster and more effectively than those who lack faith.[3] They live in a universe that is ruled by a benevolent, omnipotent God, who cares about all creation, answers their prayers, performs miracles, and offers unlimited grace to the faithful. In such a world, every life event has purpose and meaning, even a negative development such as an illness or financial problems. The religious person is capable of transforming the worst situations into positive experiences. To the faithful, seemingly simple natural events such as the changing of the seasons are experienced with awe, thankfulness, and joy as gifts from a loving Creator.

Consider the lives of Marguerite and Walter Grounds, a North Carolina couple now in their eighties, who have used their deep faith to overcome the burdens of childhood poverty, hard times in adulthood, and physical illness. They remain as cheerful and optimistic today as they were at the start of their long marriage.

Living with Optimism: Marguerite and Walter's Story

On a bright Saturday afternoon in November 1949, Walter Grounds, then a Florida railroad worker, and his wife, Marguerite, were in the kitchen of their small Miami, Florida, bungalow preparing supper. Around five, their children, Janet and Charles, returned from a matinee movie.

"Daddy," Janet, fourteen, said, "I feel real bad."

Marguerite dried her hands on a dish towel and felt the girl's flushed forehead. "She's burning up," she told her husband.

By Monday morning, Janet's fever had not broken and her joints were knotted in pain.

"Looks like a nasty bout of flu," their doctor told Walter and Marguerite.

Walter did not have the courage to voice his anxious suspicion: Miami's neighborhoods, as so much of the country, had been ravaged that summer by a terrifying polio epidemic. But so far, their children had been spared. Now he could only hope the doctor's diagnosis was accurate. Near midnight, however, his silent dread became reality. Janet lay in bed, gasping, her arms and legs stiff and useless. The next day, Walter and Marguerite watched stricken at the hospital as their sandy-haired little girl was slid into the gleaming cylinder of an iron lung.

"I have to tell you that her condition is grave," the exhausted polio ward physician told the Groundses. The paralysis had not only seized her limbs and diaphragm, but was also progressing through her abdominal nerves and muscles. Few children in her condition survived.

After feeble efforts to comfort Janet, Walter slumped down to sit on a concrete flower box just outside the wide screen window of the ward, listening to the dreadful hiss and clank of the iron lungs inside.

"Don't worry, Daddy," Janet called through the screen. "I'll be back home with you and Mama pretty soon."

Her voice broke loose a sudden and unexpected cascade of hope in Walter. "Yes, honey," he called back, "you will. We've still got one good friend left."

Walter was overwhelmed with the certainty that God would not take their child. That night, he lay awake in the darkened bedroom, softly repeating the 23rd Psalm. Each time he finished the ancient prayer, he felt a new surge of optimism. "Yea, though I walk through the valley of the shadow of death, I will fear no evil. . . ." He was not praying for himself, but for Janet, who was still too young to understand, as he did, that a person could speak directly to God and be heard. *The Lord will heal my little girl.* Birds were chirping in the warm Florida dawn when Walter finally slept, the words of the psalm still echoing in his mind.

Walter Grounds's religious faith was not the product of a traditional churchgoing, two-parent family. Raised by his grandmother in the hardscrabble hills of West Virginia, Walter had known the hunger and anguish of the Appalachian coal-mining valleys as a child. With only hand-me-down overalls and boots lined with cardboard to wear, Walter had not been a regular at the local church.

But by age nine, he had embarked on his personal religious quest. Barely old enough to read the family Bible, Walter became intrigued to learn that Jesus Christ had virtually dictated the Lord's Prayer to his disciples during the Sermon on the Mount. Walter soon acquired the habit of repetitive prayer. Each Monday he recited the Lord's Prayer at bedtime. The next night he said the prayer twice; three times on the third night; until Sunday, when he slowly, devoutly repeated the prayer seven times. Throughout his childhood and adolescence, as his family was battered by epidemics of deadly influenza, black lung disease, and the tragic accidents then so familiar to coal miners, Walter used repetitive prayer to preserve his inner peace. This practice, and his tight-knit family, helped shield him from the emotional turmoil that drove many young neighbors toward alcohol abuse.

Young Walter Grounds had no way of knowing that he had adopted one of the most effective "tactics" of emotional protection studied by psychologists. Decades later, pioneering research led by Harvard's Herbert Benson, M.D., showed that repetitive prayer and nonreligious meditation have similar relaxation effects, but that people find more emotional comfort in prayer. Repetitive prayer slows a person's heart and breathing rate, lowers blood pressure, and even calms brain waves, all without drugs. Many researchers have since studied possible biological mechanisms involved in the calming that results from meditation and prayer.[4] Walter Grounds, like many others, had come to believe as a child that God could heal emotional stress and physical illness when petitioned to do so through prayer.

And that belief was reinforced in the fall of 1949, as Janet lay in the heartbreaking grip of the iron lung. Even though her doctors remained somber and guarded in their prognosis, Walter convinced both Marguerite and their little girl that she would recover. Then, after Thanksgiving, Janet slowly began to regain neuromuscular control. She was out of the iron lung before Christmas, and home after the New Year.

As Janet continued her painful recuperation, Walter was filled with grateful joy. But he was not surprised. He *knew* that God had answered his prayers. In the coming months, Janet's recovery continued. She went back to school and responded well to physical therapy. Walter would never forget coming home from the rail yard one warm spring afternoon to find Janet sitting happily at the book-strewn kitchen table, helping her brother Charlie with his multiplication tables. Although her right leg was still supported by a brace, the girl had almost completely recovered. "When you speak directly to the Lord," he told Marguerite, "He always listens." Ironically, Walter recalls the anxious winter of Janet's illness with warm gratitude. It was then he first experienced the unbreakable personal bond to God, on whom he would rely for strength the rest of his life.

As I've already emphasized, neither I nor any other physician or scientist can validate that Janet Grounds's recovery was a miraculous cure due to divine intervention. Such spontaneous healing would be a supernatural event beyond the investigative reach of science. But Walter and Marguerite Grounds did not need such rational verification. Walter in particular became unshakably convinced that he had spoken directly to God, who had then interceded to heal their child. That conviction bolstered his already solid faith. Since those frightening weeks in 1949, Walter has remained certain that God will always remain a partner in his family's life.

Walter's work with the Seaboard Railroad took their family throughout the Southeast over the coming years before they finally settled in North Carolina. Although they attended several churches, the Groundses found their true spiritual "home" in Cheek Height Baptist Church near Durham, which they joined in 1968.

✳

The Power of "Intrinsic Religiosity"

Walter and Marguerite's faith contains obvious elements of what personality and social psychologist Gordon Allport identified as "intrinsic religiosity" in a series of pioneering studies dating back to 1950.[5] Allport, a Harvard professor who became world-renowned for his work on religious prejudice, basically divided people's faith into intrinsic and extrinsic religiosity. He found that "extrinsics" used religion to obtain some nonspiritual goal, such as finding friends or achieving social status, prestige, or power. (Think of Dana Carvey's hilarious Church Lady on *Saturday Night Live*.) But Allport found that people with deep inner ("intrinsic") faith were religious for religion's sake. This strong faith was the principal motivating force in their lives. Their faith affected their everyday behavior and decisions, and was characterized by a close personal relationship with God. To separate out the intrinsics from the extrinsics, Allport developed a twenty-item religious attitude scale.

Catholic University's Dr. Dean Hoge later modified Allport's scale to ten items that focused on the intrinsically religious. We used this shorter scale in a study I led on the connection between faith and morale among elderly Midwesterners, in which they answered questionnaires about their religion and sense of well-being. To ensure that these questions were actually measuring a personal sense of faith, we tested the Hoge scale on eighty-five ministers, priests, and rabbis. As expected, these clergy scored very high on the scale, confirming its usefulness for our study.

We found strong evidence that intrinsic religiosity (such as Walter Grounds's) was a stronger factor than social status or financial security in determining elderly people's self-perceived well-being and life satisfaction. We analyzed responses from 836 people, who included members of conservative Protestant churches, participants in a Jewish senior citizens lunch program, and almost 200 retired Dominican and Franciscan nuns. Persons scoring high on intrinsic religiosity—those who attended religious services frequently and those who prayed or read the Bible often—scored significantly higher on overall morale than the others. We concluded that religious faith was directly related to the morale and life satisfaction of elderly people, particularly women over the age of seventy-five. And this finding was not affected by people's physical health, the social support they felt from the community, or their financial status.[6]

So I was not surprised to learn that Marguerite and Walter Grounds still enjoy high morale and project an inspiring sense of life satisfaction as they prepare to celebrate their sixty-second wedding anniversary. Walter is now eighty-two, but is still robust, energetic, and optimistic. He has finally put aside a series of post-retirement jobs and devotes himself to his wife, his church, and his woodworking shop. For years, Walter was a key figure in Cheek Height Baptist Church's elaborate annual Christmas pageant, at which he was a popular narrator of the choir's cantatas. He has also been active visiting sick and shut-in church members.

"The Lord guides me in everything I do," he says simply, explaining his generosity toward others.

Marguerite, eighty-one, worked in a hospital for almost thirty years after their children grew up. She remains stubbornly cheerful despite severe health problems in recent years. Due to osteoporosis, she suffered a broken hip in 1994, and has endured major orthopedic surgery twice. She has also suffered three serious pneumonia attacks during this period.

I have treated elderly patients who have been almost emotionally crippled by depression from similar ordeals. But Marguerite Grounds relies on prayer and her husband's ongoing emotional support when pain or the frustration of immobility intrude with a temporary bout of "the blues." Commenting gratefully on the skillful medical care she has received, Marguerite says with obvious sincerity, "The Lord gave my doctors the knowledge to help me."

Coping with the Burdens of the Elderly

Marguerite and Walter Grounds are not unusual in the morale-boosting strength they draw from their faith and religious practice, as has been demonstrated by a growing body of research. In the mid-1980s, I worked with colleagues on a survey of Midwestern elderly people, attempting to determine how their religion helped them cope with the inevitable physical and emotional burdens of later life. We chose a group of outpatients attending a geriatric assessment clinic affiliated with the Southern Illinois University School of Medicine. Our study examined the religious beliefs, religious background, knowledge of scripture, importance of prayer, use of religion to cope with stress, intrinsic religiosity, and social support derived from their religious community.

Almost all the people we studied combined traditional church attendance and worship with intrinsic religious faith. More than half attended religious service at least once a week. Almost three-quarters prayed privately once or more daily. About half read religious material such as scriptural and devotional texts several times a week. Exactly 52 percent of our sample reported that most of their closest friends came from their church congregation. These people called prayer an important part of their lives, and 70 percent felt strongly they had personally experienced God's love and care. Almost two-thirds believed their relationship with God prevented loneliness, while a full 66 percent were convinced people should seek divine guidance before making any important decision.

Significantly, we found that the levels of religious practice and intrinsic faith were generally lower in patients with cancer, chronic anxiety, and measurable depression, and among people who smoked tobacco and regularly drank alcohol. This finding sparked my curiosity. Did these health factors cause people's faith to wane? Or did their relatively weaker faith somehow contribute to their other problems? I would later conduct extensive research to determine how religious faith and membership in a congregation may actually shield people from immoderate habits, emotional illness, and an impaired immune system.

In this study, after putting all the geriatric outpatient survey information through rigid statistical analysis, we reached the conclusion that religious faith, level of intrinsic religiosity, and worship patterns such as church attendance were important parts of these people's lives and probably contributed to their improved emotional and physical health.[7]

Training in family medicine in Missouri and Illinois, I often treated elderly patients similar to those in this study. Again, it was meeting people such as Ruby and Bill Clevenger and Mrs. Edna Hanson that began to shift my professional interest toward the connection between faith and health. But in retrospect, there were many older Midwesterners who impressed me with their cheerful, often intrepid good morale in later life. I can still see their weathered faces in the snowy twilight of hospital bus stops, men and women who had been battered by hard lives but who drew the courage to persevere largely from their intrinsic faith.

They had come of age in the Great Depression. Many endured years of unemployment, vainly searching for jobs with decent wages. Walter Grounds, for example, was laid off in the 1930s and had to take his young family back to West Virginia, where he mined coal in an uncle's dangerous, unlicensed claim shaft. He hacked at the coal seam with a pickax ten hours a day, and earned about one dollar, enough to buy cornmeal and dried beans, a meager supplement to the county-welfare canned beef and powdered milk. For people Walter's age, the harsh Depression lasted until the hazards, sacrifices, and anxious separations from loved ones of World War II. Yet they still truly believe God has graced their lives.

I don't want to romanticize these older people. But I often feel we who were born into the prosperous postwar world should consider the deep roots of our parents' religious beliefs. As a psychiatrist, I recognize the immense emotional support such faith provided a generation that faced a virtual twentieth-century trial of Job during the 1930s and 1940s. Ironically, these older people's faith, tempered in the crucible of the Depression and war, might actually help shield them from emotional and physical problems better than the less traditional and more questioning spiritual beliefs of their children and grandchildren. However, as we in the Baby Boom pass through middle age ourselves, we may turn in larger numbers to the faith that nurtured older generations of our families. And, in doing so, we may find greater satisfaction in later life.

Another good example of life satisfaction engendered by a sense of God's purpose in life can be found in the story of three elderly sisters from Milwaukee.

It's Never Too Late: The Story of the Three Sisters

On a recent winter Tuesday morning, Helen Koebert, eighty-two, rose at dawn and gazed out the kitchen window, frowning at the crusted snowdrifts on the lawn of the old frame house on Fernwood Avenue in Bay View, an established middle-class neighborhood on the south side of Milwaukee. The television weatherman warned of more snow, followed by intense cold. Many people Helen's age would have turned up the thermostat, pulled on a thick cardigan, and stayed indoors. Indeed, Helen was tired on this bleak winter morning, but she had responsibilities. Before fixing herself breakfast, she read a quiet meditation from *Portals of Prayer*, as was her daily habit. After eating, she dressed in storm boots and her insulated winter coat and leaned into the raw wind off Lake Michigan, negotiating the two blocks of icy sidewalk to Messiah Evangelical Lutheran Church.

She reached the church preschool well before eight, ahead of the morning "rush hour." Soon a throng of children and parents crowded the entrance. The little students ranged from sleepy three-year-olds bundled in snowsuits to some boisterous boys of five, suddenly shy as they kissed their mothers good-bye in public. Helen joined her sisters, Lorraine Kummers, eighty-three, and Esther Hart, who had just celebrated her eightieth birthday. The three exchanged greetings with Messiah Preschool director Connie Kozlowski and set to work helping the smaller children out of their parkas and making sure no mittens went astray.

The noise level in the big tile-floor classroom echoed near the pain threshold, but Helen and her sisters didn't flinch. As the children settled down in their chairs, the three white-haired sisters took their places among them, waiting for Connie to lead the morning prayer. The rest of the day melded into a predictable pattern of songs, games, and problem solving. Helen answered plaintive yelps when someone's favorite purple dinosaur was misappropriated. Lorraine supervised a quiet group of older children, bent in concentration around the puzzle table. Helen, Lorraine, and Esther, who had raised eight children among them decades earlier, and who had cared for their last toddler grandchildren in the 1980s, took turns escorting little boys and girls to the lavatory and supervising at the hand-washing sink.

But they were much more than baby-sitters. In 1994, after serving as volunteer teachers at the church, the three had enrolled at Milwaukee Area Technical College, in a class with young women their grandchildren's age, to become certified preschool teachers.

"Going back to the classroom at our age wasn't easy," Helen recalls. "But we knew Connie and the church really needed us."

Since receiving their state teaching certification, the sisters have worked five mornings and three afternoons a week. Their attendance has been excellent, even though Lorraine suffers from arthritis and osteoporosis. Each morning, winter and summer, they arrive from their nearby homes to begin another hectic, but satisfying, day among the children. "We do it for the church," Helen says, noting that her whole family was baptized, confirmed, and married in the "old" white pine-plank church with the pointy steeple, the predecessor of the newer brick building. All the children remained in Bay View. Over the decades, they have seen neighborhood streets transformed from lumpy cobblestone laced with streetcar tracks to wide asphalt lanes crowded with minivans. But, even though Messiah Church moved to a newer building a few blocks from the original site, its sustaining presence remained unchanged.

The lives of these three women, however, have had more substance and complexity than the Norman Rockwell facade many people see. "We were real poor as kids," Helen says, "at least financially."

Their father, the janitor of nearby Fernwood School, died in the 1920s, when Lorraine, the oldest, was just fourteen. His death left their mother, Emma Beyer, to raise five children on her own. She cleaned part-time at the school, took in ironing, and measured out every can of tomatoes and spoonful of macaroni. The days began and ended with prayer. Each meal, often just a bowl of potato soup, opened with grace. Emma's strong faith allowed her to surmount a life of grief and work that would have crushed a weaker person. "Mama made us all finish high school," Helen remembers, "even though we could have quit early and gotten jobs to help out more at home."

Over the next decades, as the sisters married and raised their own families, Messiah Church remained the anchor of their lives. In the 1940s, Helen's marriage ended in divorce when her son James was just four. This was a time when a "broken home" was viewed as a shameful stigma. Yet Helen found love and acceptance in her family and the church. She took an unskilled assembly job at Allen-Bradley, a large electrical equipment plant, and worked her way up to supervisor before retirement. Every Sunday and each Christmas and Easter, the family gathered to fill pews at Messiah, singing the comforting old hymns, reciting the familiar liturgy.

Beginning in the 1970s, a series of tragedies battered the family. Their mother Emma, who had taught them all their self-reliant pride, slipped into helpless, burdensome dementia, no doubt an early, undiag-nosed case of Alzheimer's. Helen stoically accepted most of the heavy burden of caring for the once-resolute woman who had been so sadly transformed by the disease. But there were days and nights when even Helen's courage faltered. That was when she spoke directly to God, for-going the words of formal prayer. "I'm not going to make it without your help," she would whisper, picking up her Bible to search the scrip-ture for solace.

Then, after death finally freed their mother from her suffering, the sisters' two younger siblings, William and Bernice, died of cancer. The triple blow tested the strength of their faith. "I learned then," Helen says, "that none of us can understand God's plan for our lives. But we must accept it with love and gratitude."

That stubborn faith was again strained when one of Lorraine's grandsons, a respected and well-loved young Christian, husband, and father, was murdered in a senseless violent act at his factory.

Instead of isolating the surviving sisters in separate cells of heartbreak, these losses drove them closer to each other and their congregation. Messiah Church had always been an island of stability in their lives. Their earliest memories were of the old white church: the echoing organ, the sparkling Christmas bulbs, and the lilies at Easter.

It made sound emotional sense for the three sisters to fall back on Messiah. In turn, the church responded with loving appreciation; without the women's dedication, the preschool, which cannot easily compete for certified teachers, would not survive. These jobs are not some token contribution arranged to make three old ladies feel better. They have a solid, ongoing responsibility. "We don't go there to play shuffleboard," Helen notes proudly. "We work hard, try to do well, and know we are needed."

Helen Koebert frankly admits that she and her sisters are not immune to normal stress and the occasional bout of depression. But like so many other religious elderly people I have encountered over the years, they use their faith, including individual prayer, inspirational reading, and regular congregational worship, to keep up morale. Certainly in their case, the emotional nurturance of fulfilling daily work is a booster to overall life satisfaction.

"Religion has always been a strong part of our lives," Helen reflects. "Our work at church is a natural part of our faith."

The Value of "Old-Time" Religion

People have celebrated the Messiah Church preschool teachers as exceptional examples of selfless faith. And, without doubt, their generous contribution is grounded in religious belief. But this impressive energy and optimism are probably more widespread than most of us realize. They could have been raised in a traditional Old World immigrant enclave, an Irish neighborhood in South Boston, a Ukrainian steel town on the Monongahela, a Welsh tin-mining village in Wisconsin or Iowa, perhaps even a cluster of Japanese-American truck farms in California's Central Valley. In those traditional minisocieties, their lives might have run parallel courses. Perhaps they would be living in a protective knot of extended family homes (analogous to their Bay View neighborhood), spending each day caring for children and in devotion at the "village" church, while younger family members worked outside the home, secure in the knowledge that their families were receiving loving attention. In surviving traditional immigrant societies here, and in their analogues overseas, the elderly do not formally *retire*, but instead assume different responsibilities as they age, their important contributions considered natural.

Does this comparison hold true for the Milwaukee sisters? I see their stable, family-oriented neighborhood, with an established church at its heart, as being similar to many traditional European or even Japanese villages. Personal (intrinsic) faith as well as congregational worship seem to be important factors in both the emotional and physical health of these communities, and probably account for much of the sisters' irrepressible energy and positive attitude.

And we now recognize that life satisfaction and good morale provide us with much more than mere emotional comfort. An overall positive attitude can influence people's physical health and even their longevity in several ways. People who face life with an optimistic sense of purpose within God's plan pay more attention to good nutrition and moderate exercise than people with poor morale. And recent research sponsored by the U.S. Department of Health and Human Services shows that eating well and engaging in regular moderate physical activity such as walking, yard work, and housekeeping can help prevent a number of the chronic diseases of later life.[8] Elderly people like Walter Grounds and Helen Koebert, who honestly report that they "feel young," generally do show fewer negative signs of aging than people who are anxiously preoccupied with their encroaching mortality. I know as a geriatric specialist that older people with positive attitudes tend to follow their doctors' advice about diet and medication more closely than depressed elderly patients. So, on the whole, the good morale and general life satisfaction enjoyed by so many people with strong religious faith tends to reinforce the classic medical adage, "A sound mind in a sound body" (*Mens sana in corpore sano*).

Studying Morale and Religious Faith

University of Texas sociologist Christopher G. Ellison published research in 1991 that provides a compelling scientific explanation for the connection between good morale and religious faith and practice. Ellison's team studied data from the national General Social Survey, an annual random sampling of adults, most younger than sixty-five, that statistics experts value for its wide demographic base. The 1988 survey included a unique series of questions on the sociological aspects of religion, personal faith, and religious practice that were previously never asked. Ellison was particularly interested in the connection between religious belief and practice and what sociologists call "subjective well-being," another term for good morale or life satisfaction.

He investigated several variables, including the social support and the bolstering of morale and healthy behavior that many people receive from membership in church or synagogue congregations, as well as the emotional uplift of group worship. Ellison also looked into the psychological impact of deep personal faith and people's sense of connection to God, often experienced during private spiritual practices, such as individual prayer and scriptural reading. The people in the survey included conservative, moderate, liberal, and nondenominational Protestants, Roman Catholics, Jews, Mormons, and Jehovah's Witnesses.

The findings, which were derived from rigorous statistical analysis, demonstrate how religious faith and practice enhance life satisfaction. People of all ages with strong intrinsic belief had a generally better perceived quality of life than those with less fervent faith. The survey data suggested that attendance at worship service and private devotion only *indirectly* contribute to life satisfaction. But a strong personal faith directly shields people from life's inevitable problems, which in turn increases a sense of well-being. I must add here that the people in the survey ranged widely in age and social-financial status, so these findings do not just apply to elderly people who might turn to religion for comfort late in life.

Significantly, Ellison's research found that "strong religious faith makes traumatic events easier to bear."[9] This research evidence certainly helps explain how people like Marguerite Grounds and Helen Koebert and her sisters can maintain a positive attitude about life, given the problems they've had to overcome.

Further, Ellison's study demonstrated that people affiliated with a church congregation felt "significantly greater life satisfaction than unaffiliated individuals."[10] Again, I am reminded of the Groundses and the Milwaukee sisters, whose lives are centered on their churches. But this boost in positive outlook is certainly not limited to elderly white people. Indeed, the data Ellison used from the General Social Survey cut across the boundaries of age, race, and religious denomination.

African-American Faith: Khalita's Story

Jeffrey Levin, M.D., a senior research fellow at the National Institute for Healthcare Research in Rockville, Maryland, and his colleagues found confirmation that church membership and attendance supports life satisfaction among African-Americans ranging in age from eighteen to over fifty-five. Levin also presented significant evidence suggesting that membership in a predominantly African-American church congregation was associated with better overall physical health.[11]

I recently had the pleasure of meeting a young African-American woman named Khalita Jones, who embodies several of the qualities noted in this research. At our first meeting, Khalita was friendly and well-spoken, a university student who displayed an unusually mature and thoughtful manner for a person of twenty-one. But I knew from medical colleagues that she had been struggling with chronic, serious illness since childhood. I discovered that Khalita's serenity in the face of adversity was grounded in her religious faith and the support of church congregations.

Khalita Jones was born in the small town of Lexington in the North Carolina Piedmont, the second of two children. Her mother, a high school teacher, and father, who worked at Lexington Furniture Industries, were lifelong members of the local AME Zion church. Having been brought to church since infancy, Khalita tells friends that she "grew up" in the congregation.

When she was only four, her parents became alarmed at the little girl's frequent bruising and unexplained weakness. After a frustrating medical odyssey, Khalita was finally diagnosed with a nontypical form of aplastic anemia that was deemed to be autoimmune in nature. This is a life-threatening illness that presents characteristics similar to leukemia. Khalita's bone marrow does not make enough healthy red or white blood cells or platelets. Her immune system is chronically weakened, making her vulnerable to debilitating infections. Although she does quite well considering her low blood counts, Khalita has become accustomed from early childhood onward to painful, frightening, and sometimes lonely visits to the hospital.

Yet she remained active in school and church, where she sang in the choir and performed as an acolyte. When Khalita was older, she taught Sunday school and always volunteered to serve at church activities such as suppers, social events, and prayer meetings. If her illness kept her in bed, Khalita insisted on completing her schoolwork, and even on doing paperwork for church projects.

Still in adolescence, Khalita persevered during several grave crises in her life, including the intense emotional strain of balancing the physical restraints of her illness with the demands of achieving academic excellence. I've seen many young people in her position emotionally collapse under such a stressful burden. Even physically healthy teenagers often feel oppressed by the "unfair" demands of growing up. Instead, Khalita Jones undertook a spiritual quest, hoping to learn why she had been called upon to endure this suffering.

Only a high school student, she found time for both her classes and serious scriptural investigation. By age eighteen, Khalita was absolutely certain that God was testing her in a way similar to the ordeals faced by the "righteous" people in the Bible, although she understood early on that such righteousness accrues from God's grace, not personal desire. Like so many who draw strength from religious faith, Khalita firmly believed she had identified God's plan in her life: Despite her illness, God wanted her to finish high school, graduate from college, and become a

Christian guidance counselor for troubled families and youngsters.

Khalita worked with stubborn determination to follow this plan. After graduating from high school in Lexington, she enrolled as an undergraduate at Duke University, majoring in psychology. But the normal stress and fatigue of student life rekindled her illness and she was repeatedly hospitalized with infections and perilously low blood counts. Most young people facing such setbacks would have retreated. Khalita merely changed her tactics, reducing her class load and accepting incompletes when the illness kept her from finishing projects. But she stayed in school twelve months a year, doggedly making up her incompletes and fulfilling her requirements. She is now finishing her senior year.

Despite all the fear and disappointment, Khalita remains tranquil and optimistic. "I *know* God will help me when I need Him most," she says.

Further, knowing that people are concerned about her undoubtedly strengthens Khalita's morale. Since she joined a church in Durham that is very popular with Duke students, her new congregation has rallied to her side whenever Khalita is ill. Church members drive her to class and medical appointments when she is too weak to walk, help with her shopping, and often drop by with tempting meals when the side effects of medication would otherwise discourage her from eating. And she knows that the members of her "home" church in Lexington maintain an ongoing prayer vigil for her. Such tangible support shields Khalita from the emotional isolation that often accompanies chronic physical illness and underlies poor morale or an overall negative outlook.

Khalita helps maintain her cheerful attitude through spiritual discipline. She begins each morning kneeling in prayer, an overt demonstration to God that she has surrendered to His divine will. Her formal prayer always brings a physical sense of calm, which prepares her emotionally for the inevitable challenges of the day. As she communes with God during prayer, she takes a few moments to record in one of her devotional journals what God is telling her about her life.

Each noon, Khalita takes time for a private "talk with God," during which she reads scripture and seeks strength from the Lord to persevere through the rest of the day. She also writes in a devotional journal that has excerpts from inspirational writers as well as biblical text that might help her find strength.

At the end of the day, Khalita writes in another devotional journal, then kneels in prayer in submission to the Lord. She always offers thanks, despite any unpleasant side effects from her strong medications or anxiety from the uncertainty she has seen among her physicians.

"I'm not your 'bubbly' type of college girl," she admits in her thoughtful manner. "But most of the time, I am sincerely joyful. I have no real regrets."

Without question, Khalita does find joy in the emotional certainty that she has identified and is following God's plan for her life. In this regard, and despite her serious physical problems, Khalita displays a mature—or what she calls "God-given"—wisdom I have rarely seen in anyone her age.

I'm sure that Khalita Jones will maintain this fundamental sense of well-being into later life. This would be consistent with other research Dr. Jeffrey Levin conducted after his pioneering study of black congregations, investigating the relationship of religious practice to well-being among Hispanic young adults. The study found that frequent church attendance was a reliable predictor of overall well-being twelve years later.[12] And a study focusing on the relationship of religion and emotional pain among African-American women found that those with moderate or high religious faith were less likely to suffer psychological distress than those who scored low on a standard test of religiosity.[13]

Certainly, my experience as a physician and psychiatrist has taught me the critical value of positive attitude and sincere life satisfaction. Armed with this often elusive quality, people can cope much more easily with the inevitable daily stress and occasional more severe trauma that are woven into the fabric of our existence. In many people who display such life satisfaction whom I have studied, I have found a solid foundation of religious faith, which generally included the quiet but unshakable knowledge that God was actively working in their lives.

This certainty buffered them from emotional trauma as they passed along life's odyssey of joy, sadness, satisfactions, and hope.

The shield of such faith does not require religious people to stay home, isolated and out of harm's way, in order to keep belief intact. They can take chances in the uncertain marketplace; they can explore and train in exciting new technology; they can travel to and live in distant, apparently alien cities, secure in the comforting knowledge that their strongest relationships—to God and their family—will always be intact.

Chapter Three

✳

Religious People Have Stronger Marriages and Families

During years of clinical practice in family medicine and psychiatry, I have seen firsthand the suffering that accompanies broken marriages. My fellow mental health professionals will attest to the fact that much of today's widespread depression and substance abuse—involving both drugs and alcohol—has its roots in marital strife, including divorce and its inevitable emotional and social dislocation. The alarming rate of physical abuse in households, usually inflicted on women and children, almost always arises after the original bond of love and trust between a couple is shattered.

And, no matter how "friendly" or legally nonadversarial a divorce, its psychological trauma is invariably slow to heal. In fact, therapists learn that the emotional impact of a broken marriage is almost as painful as the death of a loved one. It's certainly been my experience in treating adults and young people that the emotional tempest swirling around divorce, especially when children are involved, can upset lives for years.

Is divorce really as grave a social problem as it is portrayed in the news media? Let's look at some statistics. In 1996, there were approximately 2,344,000 marriages in the United States. But there were also 1,150,000 divorces, a total that has remained relatively constant in recent years. Of course, this does not mean that half of all new marriages *will* end in divorce, but about 40 percent probably will.

In each recent year there has been an average of four million children whose lives were disrupted by divorce. This amounts to over sixty million American adults and children involved in broken homes in the 1990s alone.

Fortunately, in recent years there has also been a slow decline in the relative divorce rate, as measured by number per 1,000 total population. In 1979, for example, the per-1,000 rate was 6.3; in 1996 it dropped to 4.3; and in the first six months of 1997, the rate was hovering near that level.[1] And I have seen couples and families who were actively considering divorce able to shore up and strengthen their relationships through a combination of religious faith, marital counseling, and renewed dedication to keeping their family intact.

We could certainly use more of this dedication. Divorce statistics make it painfully clear that broken homes today are much more common than they were in earlier generations: In 1940, the per-1,000 rate was 2.0, and it had risen to only 2.2 by 1960.[2]

Divorce and the Emotional Problems of Children

My Baby Boom generation is divorcing at more than twice the rate of our parents and grandparents. And we are suffering the consequences. A few years ago, the National Center for Health Statistics compiled pioneering research on the developmental and emotional problems of American children. The study examined children living in the homes of their biological parents as well as "disrupted and reconstituted families," which included single-parent homes (often headed by divorced mothers).[3] One of the report's most significant findings: "Children in disrupted families were nearly twice as likely as those in mother-father families to have developmental, learning, or behavioral problems."[4] These contributed to higher rates of adolescent pregnancy, drug abuse, and juvenile crime than those of children living with both married parents. The authors found that the troublesome situation often persisted from infancy through adolescence, ultimately involving millions of young people, and representing a major burden for our schools, health care system, and juvenile justice authorities.

In 1993, the principal author of this report, researcher Nicholas Zill, Ph.D., and his colleagues studied the impact of divorce on young adults. They found that, largely regardless of economic or social status, young people eighteen to twenty-two years old who were children when their parents divorced "were twice as likely as other youths to have poor relationships with their fathers and mothers, to show high levels of emotional distress or problem behavior, to have received psychological help, and to have dropped out of high school at some point."[5]

This is grim evidence of a festering social wound. But can we find practical ways to keep marriages intact in our present cultural milieu, which celebrates casual sexuality and seems to honor selfishness and hedonism as virtues?

I certainly don't have all the answers. But I do know from my experience as a clinician and a researcher that religious faith often restores peace to a troubled marriage and bolsters a family during times of intense stress. There is significant evidence that couples sharing religious faith and practice will divorce less often than couples without a meaningful mutual faith. For example, data concerning white and black Protestants and white Catholics taken from a large national survey in the 1970s when the divorce wave was cresting revealed that the divorce or separation rate was 34 percent among couples attending church less than once a year, but only 18 percent for those attending monthly or more frequently. That means that the more religious people (as measured by church attendance) divorced or separated about half as often as the less religious.[6] And recent studies show that people with strong religious faith are more likely to protect their marriages as something sacred, to seek pastoral counseling, and to take steps to modify their behavior in order to prevent divorce.[7]

The Family as a Divine Social Unit

All the world's religions hold that the family is a divinely ordained social unit. Religions discourage divorce, support family reconciliation, and command us not to seek intimate relationships outside of marriage. Husband and wife are instructed to honor and respect each other and to raise their children to follow an unequivocal moral code.[8]

Research also indicates that prayer and meditation, both as individuals and as couples, is an important factor in the success of such pastoral intervention. Increasingly, the major denominations rely upon marriage-enrichment seminars, which have become a type of "preventive maintenance" for families in their congregations.[9]

Religious Marital Counseling: Ellen and Tom's Story

Practicing individual and family psychiatry, I have counseled many religious couples experiencing problems in their marriage. One couple, whom I will call Tom and Ellen, are typical of people I've treated who draw on religious faith for the strength to repair a seemingly irreconcilable situation.

Ellen and Tom had been married about ten years when a colleague referred them to me. "I wish you luck, Harold," the colleague said with a chuckle. "They're nice people, but I certainly have not been able to help them."

Indeed, Tom and Ellen had spent almost half of their ten-year marriage seeing marital counselors.

"Looks like that's all we ever do," Tom complained with an ironic grin during their first visit to my office. Then he added that their last two counselors, including my colleague, had "fired" the couple as patients.

Ellen and Tom had three young children. Tom had worked his way up to a well-paid professional position, while Ellen, also college-educated, had not been employed outside their home since marrying.

As was true of some other couples I'd encountered, Ellen and Tom had rigid and very self-centered personalities that conceivably might have meshed well in another marriage but were the source of constant tension with their existing spouses. Twenty minutes into our first session, I realized I faced a definite challenge with this couple. The intense sessions that followed confirmed my initial apprehension.

Tom was a classic workaholic. When he described his promotions and accomplishments, I realized he derived most of his self-esteem from his executive image, not from being a husband or a father. "I get along with everybody at the office," Tom insisted. "I just don't see why Ellen resents me so."

For her part, Ellen had longed to leave the hectic workplace and devote herself to being a full-time mother. But raising three children only five years apart in age had become drudgery, not the rich fulfillment she'd envisioned. One of her main complaints was that Tom made no effort to help around the house. She bitterly viewed his professional commitment as competition, and frequently begged him to spend more time with her and the children.

"I'd love to, Doctor," Tom answered with controlled indignation. "But I'm worn out when I come home, and all I get is grief." Then he grudgingly admitted that much of the "overtime" he spent at the office provided a welcome sanctuary from conflict at home.

In another session, Ellen accused Tom of being "very controlling" when he was home and criticizing her for minor housekeeping problems. Tom hotly disputed this and shot back accusations that it was Ellen who was the "control freak" because she wouldn't let him roughhouse with the children, which, he said, they loved.

Ellen, stiff with indignation, rolled her eyes, then related she found it distasteful that when Tom did find time to play with the children, he "acted like a little kid." She emphasized that small children really wanted "adult guidance" from their father.

Later sessions often skidded toward similar purposeless reciprocal vituperation, which invariably dredged up lists of hurts, some dating back years.

It became obvious that Ellen and Tom were basically antagonistic personality types, so different that I was amazed they had married in the first place and had somehow not yet divorced.

Tom's idea of a pleasant evening at home was watching violent horror films, which repulsed Ellen, who was drawn toward romantic stories. Tom insisted they put a fixed percentage of his earnings into secure savings for the future. Ellen loved to spend money on expensive clothes for the family and on stylish furniture. They disagreed on how the children should be disciplined, what and when they should eat, even on presents at Christmas and birthdays. Tom liked large, traditional meat-and-potatoes meals, while Ellen preferred lighter, near-vegetarian food.

"What about religion?" I asked. "Do you agree about spiritual matters?"

They looked surprised. "Sure," Tom said with a shrug.

"Of course," Ellen added.

We'll see, I thought, jotting a note.

As it turned out, they did seem to share an abiding faith in God. But Ellen loved the ceremony, ritual, and social pleasantries of church services, while Tom felt uncomfortable at these functions and preferred to spend precious weekend time camping and boating with the children. For Tom, the seemingly endless "chitchat" at church coffees was painful, reminding him of the hours he spent each week with clients. But Ellen reveled in church social life, as long as she had her successful, well-dressed husband and attractive children at her side.

"Haven't you ever tried to talk these problems out?" I asked.

They both replied frankly that in recent years their level of communication had dwindled to a nonthreatening minimum out of fear of upsetting each other. Naturally, their sex life had deteriorated. I could see how they'd reached this tense standoff, so typical among couples on the verge of divorce. Stress is part of the daily lives of such bright high achievers. Tom wanted a dazzling business career and the warmly supportive family he thought automatically came with that success. Ellen was convinced that her family had to display each of the traditional attributes of happiness and prosperity, from spotless soccer jerseys to a handsome husband in an expensive new suit standing beside her in church each Sunday.

But confronted by the stressful reality of their lives, as opposed to their immature ideals, they vented irritation and withdrew from each other. This, of course, set in motion a wheel of negative emotional feedback that only increased their stress levels.

Although both claimed the habit of daily prayer, at this troubled point in their lives they were unable to enjoy the stress-reducing inner comfort of that prayer because they were choked with resentment toward each other. I tried to gently assess their true level of faith and was mildly surprised to find that each had a firm belief in God that had remained unshaken since childhood. And they both convincingly stated that for them, marriage was a sacred commitment, despite their blatant conflicts. Separately, they each voiced their love for the other and vowed to remain in counseling indefinitely if that would help their marriage.

One of Ellen's spontaneous declarations gave me hope. "I believe that God can help work things out," she told me earnestly, "either by helping me change, or by helping Tom."

That was a major admission for a person who was just as rigid as her husband. I had already concluded that they were both so immature and self-centered that neither seemed likely to accept the painful work of personal compromise required to enable them to grow as a healthy couple. But they surprised me. I had available the standard arsenal of marital counselor's tools, which began with simple cooperative "homework" exercises leading toward more important compromises. But other counselors had failed with this repertoire. So I decided to frame *every* suggestion, each communication exercise and weekly cooperative checklist item within a Christian context. In a sense, I briefly became Ellen and Tom's spiritual adviser as well as their counselor.

To my surprise, the couple began to change. As long as I stressed that the God-ordained sanctity of their marriage required them to work toward better cooperation, become more flexible, and to practice more open communication, Tom and Ellen responded. Whenever I made equally logical suggestions outside a religious context, they ignored me, as they had so many other marriage counselors. That was okay. I don't have a fragile ego when it comes to results.

Six months later, Tom and Ellen were making amazing progress. Tom was beginning to grasp that, in a religious marriage, a husband and father should be an active participant in home life, not simply a dependable provider. Because his low self-esteem had been bolstered by the accolades that accompanied his business success for so long, however, Tom was slow to change his workaholic habits. But he did eventually adjust his schedule. Finding himself at home more often in the afternoon, he saw the hectic challenge Ellen had faced alone— fixing the children's dinner, supervising their homework, and then preparing the elaborate traditional "home cooking" he expected as his due each evening. He realized that it was his duty as a religiously committed partner in this marriage to pitch in with these chores.

For her part, Ellen gradually accepted the unpleasant reality that the social veneer of a prosperous, contented home could be a facade hiding an empty relationship. Dressing her husband, herself, and their children in expensive clothes, then parading them through endless hours of church social life, had been, in fact, the attempt of an immature person to seek attention. With Tom home early each day, she forced herself to allow Tom a normal period of healthy roughhousing with the children, even though this play inevitably sent her meticulously (and obsessively) arranged cushions and throw rugs asunder.

I'll not try to sugarcoat this account by claiming the first months of Ellen and Tom's reconciliation were peaceful. In fact, forced to confront their own shortcomings, they often lashed out angrily. But the shock of these bitter encounters made them reflect on the religious faith that was the foundation of their struggle to save their marriage. For the first time, Tom and Ellen began to pray together for guidance.

A year after we met, I was confident that their marriage would survive. And I was also heartened to realize that, as individuals, they were grappling with their selfish immaturity. A colleague asked me whether it was wise for two such different personalities to remain married. And I replied honestly: "You'd be surprised. They're not the same people you tried to counsel."

I think the best demonstration that Ellen and Tom have found practical means to work together toward a healthier relationship can be found in their new patterns of religious practice. On most Sundays, they attend church together, but Ellen resists dressing her family as if they were posing for a ladies' magazine photo shoot. They keep the after-service socializing to a polite minimum. Then they "hit the trail," as Tom puts it, spending the rest of the Sunday pursuing the outdoor activities Tom loves so much.

Some mental health professionals would argue that it would have been better for a couple like Tom and Ellen to make a clean split and try to find more compatible partners in new marriages. I answer this argument by citing research on the almost inevitable emotional trauma divorce inflicts on children. I also point out that Tom and Ellen's shared religious commitment gave them the strength to work toward emotional maturity. Had they simply divorced and remarried, they probably would have experienced the same type of conflict with their new spouses that had plagued the first ten years of their relationship. But today, both have told me they feel a deep satisfaction in their life together that they never would have thought possible. In fact, Tom recently paid his wife what I consider the ultimate compliment: "If I had it to do all over again, I'd marry her tomorrow."

Religion and Marital Harmony

Is Tom and Ellen's success relevant to the current epidemic of divorce? A growing body of scientific evidence on the relationship between religion and marital harmony suggests that their achievement can be emulated by other couples who share a strong bond of faith. For example, twenty years ago sociologists Philip R. Kunz and Stan L. Albrecht found that couples who regularly practiced a common religion had a high degree of marital stability. Significantly, the regular church attenders surveyed were more likely to "select the same spouse over again" than nonattenders. And 83 percent of the regular church attenders in the survey reported they were still married to their first spouse, which was a high percentage for the socially turbulent 1970s when the Baby Boomers were reaching full adulthood.[10]

Later research that focused on one rural and one urban Kansas community reached similar findings. Both in the small town and the city, marital happiness was closely correlated with a personal sense of religious faith, which was separate from the positive social aspects of religious practice derived from church attendance.[11]

A Troubled Jewish Marriage: Dan and Marcia's Story

I want to emphasize that achieving reconciliation in a troubled marriage through renewal of religious faith is not unique to Christianity.

There is a long tradition of rabbinical spiritual advice to the individual in Judaism; in fact, much of the moral grounding of Western family life is anchored in the Torah, as well as the New Testament. And spiritually based marital counseling is slowly beginning to grow among Jewish congregations in America. Certainly Judaism provides believers a rich, emotionally nurturing faith that can help bolster commitment during serious marital problems. I think the following story of a couple in their thirties, whom I'll call Dan and Marcia, offers a moving example of the power of faith to heal a seemingly irreparable breach.

Although both Dan and Marcia had received some religious training as children, they only worshiped when their families gathered on High Holidays. Ironically, Dan, raised in a Reform family, felt vaguely drawn to the rich liturgy and mysticism of Orthodox Judaism. And Marcia, whose father had been a member of an Orthodox congregation, was attracted to the progressive intellectual attitude she found in Dan's home.

The couple bought a comfortable suburban home after Dan completed graduate school and took a position with a prestigious East Coast company. Dan, whose family had struggled running a small business, was desperate to become an executive as quickly as possible. This meant devoting all his intelligence and energy to work. Marcia found herself increasingly isolated with their infant son in the prosperous confines of their home. Dan's daily schedule often kept him in the city from early morning until near midnight. Unlike other young fathers, Dan volunteered for weekend projects and business trips, often at the last moment. Although Dan advanced much faster than his peers, Marcia's isolation deepened. Her resolution to lose the extra pounds she had gained in pregnancy faltered. Food dominated her life, and she became seriously overweight.

Dan held up well to his self-imposed demanding professional strain until an unexpected trip stranded him out of state, working all weekend on an urgent project. Then he gave in to a brief fling with a woman from another branch of the company. But he was wrought by guilt as he watched Marcia struggle with her weight. With this anguish inside him, Dan decided he must confess his infidelity. One night after dinner, he blurted out his admission. This was poor judgment. Her latest diet plan a failure, Marcia's self-image was very low, her emotional vulnerability extreme. When Dan revealed that he had been "unfaithful" on one of his business trips, Marcia reacted with jealous outrage. She obsessively searched out the woman's picture in the company's employee magazine, and was crushed to find that her rival was a slender, fashionably dressed young executive.

For hours that awful night, the couple traded hateful insults, screaming loud enough to terrify their little son. Marcia claimed that the only reason Dan had ever worked such long hours was to spend time with "sluts." Bitterly hurt that she would dismiss his exhausting years on the corporate treadmill, Dan snapped that her distasteful obesity had driven him to "other women." They both recognized the absurdity of these cruel accusations, but neither would retract or apologize.

Crushed by Dan's anger, Marcia demanded that he leave the house. The next afternoon, he found himself banished to the city, staring woodenly at hastily packed suitcases on the floor of a rented studio apartment near his office.

"What's happened to my life?" he moaned, trying to gauge the full scope of his situation. The cramped room was suddenly impossible to bear. Dan ripped open his suitcases, found a pair of sneakers, then fled the building and strode toward a nearby park. He trudged through the humid summer afternoon down a side street that was strangely crowded with men. *What the hell is this,* he thought irritably, *some kind of parade?* Then he saw that many of the men wore yarmulkes. They were Jews on their way to a nearby synagogue. "It's Friday," he muttered, "the Sabbath."

Dan surrendered to the impulse to join the throng of worshipers inside. As the cantor's melodic voice echoed from the vaulted ceiling, Dan hung back near the entrance, swept with conflicting emotions. He wanted to pray with the congregation, singing the ancient Hebrew liturgy he had rarely heard since his bar mitzvah almost twenty years before. But he felt tainted, an impostor. Dan stayed half hidden at the rear of the synagogue for the entire service. Outside in the summer twilight, he still felt alone among the men of the congregation. He was hungry, but found the prospect of taking a carry-out dinner to his office and working late depressing. Then a young man approached him with a tentative smile.

"Are you from out of town?" the stranger asked.

Dan was embarrassed. "Yeah," he said. "I guess I am."

The young man invited Dan to share the first Sabbath meal with his family. "Beats greasy egg foo young in a carton," Dan conceded, an attempt at wit that failed with this religious young man.

The man insisted they take a bus to his apartment, even though Dan offered to pay the taxi fare. A fallen-away Jew might be driving the cab, the man cautioned, and riding with him on Shabbat would be abetting his sin. Dan bit back an ironic rejoinder, realizing the man followed the more rigorous doctrines of Judaism that forbade any type of work on the Sabbath.

Dan was moved when he met the family around the Sabbath table. The eldest daughter, a girl about ten, proudly announced that she and her mother had lit the candles "exactly" at the prescribed hour. The cup of wine, the prayers chanted in the son's piping voice, above all the guileless love bonding the couple and their three children, sparked a desolate longing in Dan. Before marrying Marcia, he had daydreamed about just this type of family dinner—absent, of course, the candlesticks, the prayers, and the table laden with kosher food.

More prayers followed the meal. Then the children were excused to play on the wedge of grass behind the building. Dan's friend suggested a walk on the cooling sidewalks before dark. As they strolled the old neighborhood, where Hispanic bodegas crowded the surviving kosher shops, Dan opened up and slowly related the circumstances that had brought him to the city.

His new friend listened with a concerned frown. "At least it's good that you came back to Temple" was his only comment.

That night in the stuffy little apartment, Dan fought the temptation to call Marcia. He slept badly and awoke to a cloudy Saturday and deserted city streets. Unable to concentrate on work, Dan walked hesitantly toward the synagogue.

In the cloying afternoon heat, he bowed his head with the men around him and heard the rabbi chant a memorial prayer for a member of the congregation: "*Ha-Makom yenahem etkhembetokh*. . . ."—"May the All-and-Ever-Present comfort you. . . ."

As the men joined the timeless kaddish, Dan was inexplicably certain that they were granting him comfort and absolution for what he considered his unforgivable acts. He was stunned to actually feel a cramping weight slip from his neck and shoulders. Later, as he stood alone in the synagogue vestibule, quietly sobbing, a well-dressed older man led Dan outside. The man was connected with a Jewish counseling center. "I think you could use someone to talk with," he suggested.

Based on this unexpected emotional catharsis, Dan, the savvy, hard-headed executive, further surprised himself by opting for a rabbinical counselor, not a secular therapist.

A week later, Marcia reluctantly accepted the counseling rabbi's invitation to meet Dan at the center to explore the possibility of reconciliation. Encouraged by the rabbi, they forgave each other for any act or omission that had strained their marriage. Then the couple embarked on a year of intense rabbinical counseling.

In those twelve months, both Dan and Marcia came to recognize the spiritual void at the center of their lives. Once Dan forced himself to change his compulsive work habits, he began to realize that he could lead a normal professional life and still be a good husband and father. The couple joined a suburban synagogue and enrolled their son in weekly religious classes.

Marcia now decided to keep a kosher home and to observe the traditional Sabbath. She also entered a women's exercise and diet program sponsored by the synagogue, which emphasized small portions and the spiritual significance of traditional foods. Through this innovative program, Marcia has begun to shift her attitude about eating and now feels a sense of control over food rather than being victimized by its addictive power, as she had been for years.

To demonstrate his renewed dedication to his family, Dan now keeps every Friday afternoon free to practice his faith. No matter the press of business, he leaves the office in time to reach the family's synagogue for Sabbath service. After every Friday's services, he and Marcia are always at the table with their son, saying the first prayer in the light of the Sabbath candles.

It would be nice if I could report that their return to faith has solved all of Dan and Marcia's problems. But that would be simplistic. As we've seen with Ellen and Tom, however, faith can give people the strength to search themselves for negative attitudes and harmful patterns of behavior and can provide the motivation and strength needed to correct them. Certainly Marcia and Dan's renewed faith has helped them accept each other as flawed, but potentially better human beings.

Recently Dan told his rabbinical counselor, "Returning to Judaism has given meaning to my life and structure to my family."

Religion helped Dan and Marcia confront stress and reduced the emotional torment they were suffering. But can their embracing of Judaism provide the lasting support their marriage will require?

There is convincing evidence suggesting Judaism can provide just such a buttress. In a thorough, multiyear comparison of religion and health at secular and religious kibbutzim in Israel, researchers found "highly stable marital bonding" among the religious couples studied. Even though the kibbutz as an institution was found to be a "close-knit, family-oriented society," the divorce rate at secular kibbutzim was eleven times higher than at their religious counterparts. Further, researchers identified a stronger sense of overall well-being among the religious Jews they studied compared to their secular peers.[12]

Commenting on the role of faith in reconciliations such as Dan and Marcia's, Rabbi Simkah Weintraub of the Jewish Healing Center in New York cited an especially relevant maxim by the nineteenth-century writer who used the pen name Ahad HaAm ("One of the People"): "More than Israel [the Jewish people] has kept the Sabbath, the Sabbath has kept Israel."

A Test of Faith: Pat and Lois's Story

Confronting the emotional aftermath of infidelity was just as harsh a challenge to Dan and Marcia's marriage as the chronic personality conflict that Ellen and Tom faced. But sometimes marital stress comes from external events, such as those that afflicted Pat and Lois Cox.

It was the missionary zeal of an evangelical campus ministry that brought Pat and Lois together in the late 1970s. After their marriage in 1980, they continued working at an Alabama campus mission and lived frugally on part-time wages.

But the financial strain began to mount when Lois became pregnant with their first daughter. Pat took the traditional view that the husband should control the family checkbook. Lois found this acceptable, provided they had enough money to meet what she considered minimum standards. She was certainly not extravagant and did not object to small apartments in run-down neighborhoods, nor to plain food and inexpensive clothing; both she and Pat found their basic fulfillment in their evangelical missionary work.

This relative happiness was battered three years later, however, by a life-threatening medical crisis. They were working on a North Carolina campus in 1983 when Pat returned to their crowded little flat early one afternoon and slumped at the kitchen table, shielding his head in his hands. "This headache is just something else," he said, sighing. "I've taken a handful of aspirin already and it hasn't even put a dent in it."

Lois was hurrying to feed and bathe their toddler, Kristin, before rushing off to her part-time job. "Are you going to be okay with the baby?" she asked anxiously.

"I just don't know," Pat admitted.

Over the next three months, Lois experienced fear unlike any she had known. Pat normally enjoyed exuberant good health. But in the coming weeks his headaches grew into a constant agony. As members of their church rallied around the young couple with emotional support and prayer, Lois finally persuaded Pat to see a doctor. He was evaluated at the local medical school. An MRI scan confirmed a large dark mass in a ventricle deep within the fragile recesses of Pat's brain. Staring at the milky images of the scan, Lois listened numbly as the neurosurgeon described a potentially life-threatening colloid cyst that was causing excruciating internal brain pressure. Only invasive surgery could drain the cyst. Lois sat immobile, verging between denial and panic as the doctor droned on.

Driving home in their old sedan, Pat slumped in the passenger seat, shading his eyes from the Carolina sun while trying to renew his optimism. "God will bring a miracle," he said. "They won't have to operate." However, the surgery proved necessary to save his life. Two weeks later, the doctor pronounced the operation successful and released Pat from the hospital. But Lois quickly noticed that the young man who returned home was subtly different from the one she had married. Although Pat soon regained his mobility and dexterity, his mental acuity was altered and his basic attitudes had shifted.

One of Pat's most attractive attributes had been his love for music. He could play several instruments and had joyfully led ministry choirs. Now music meant nothing to him, and he ignored the work of students he had been coaching. Worse, his short-term memory was badly eroded. He forgot appointments, addresses and telephone numbers, and simple household tasks. Lois had always playfully chided Pat for being a "health-food nut." Now he gorged himself on candy and junk-food snacks.

After several months of this deterioration, Lois sought out Pat's doctors. "He's just not the same," she explained.

One of the physicians upbraided her. "You should be happy he's alive."

But living with Pat was not a happy experience. His neurological damage undercut his ability to make long-term plans. When Lois spoke of job openings or finding a better apartment, Pat stared at her with little apparent interest. "Okay, sure," he would always reply, but rarely followed up on her advice. Slowly, Lois came to realize Pat's personality had been altered in the aftermath of the surgery. Lethargy had replaced his previous energetic optimism. His horizons seemed to have narrowed. Even though he remained relatively fit and youthful, it was as if an older, duller person was now inhabiting his body.

The warm bond of affection they had shared chilled over the next few years. They were no longer the enthusiastic young missionary couple eager to spread the Good News gospel on college campuses. Lois's faith remained strong, and she realized that beneath his burden of postoperative brain trauma, Pat was struggling to keep his faith active.

Pat and Lois continued to pray together as they had throughout their marriage. Now Lois suggested that they ask God to bring them the strength to overcome this health crisis. It was hard for her to judge the impact of this prayer on Pat, but she did feel a growing infusion of emotional certainty in him, which she identified with divine grace. "God has a plan for our marriage," she reassured Pat.

Lois embarked on an odyssey of spiritual exploration based on scriptural and other devotional reading, helped by prayer counselors at their new evangelical church. One doctrine she discovered in this quest would become a central theme in her life and marriage: "Being a Christian means working to develop the character of Christ." Lois would need that strength in the years that lay ahead.

Through stubborn determination, Pat was eventually able to overcome his worst neurological deficits and became a route driver for a national courier service. This was an amazing achievement for someone who had trouble remembering simple number or word sequences. But although his job helped restore some of Pat's innate optimism, his long-term planning abilities were slow to return. And because Pat still managed the couple's household budget, they constantly found themselves overspent, harassed by bill collectors.

On many occasions during this period, Lois lashed out angrily, as much in self-pity as in rage at Pat's frustrating condition. It would have been easy to walk out the door with Kristin and her little sister Sarah and try to find a husband who could provide a more normal home. But every time Lois was tempted to do so, she prayed for guidance. And the calm inner voice she always heard during prayer reminded her that marriage was a sacred commitment and that these hard times would eventually end. This emotional underpinning allowed her to continue in the marriage and to make sacrifices a less spiritual person might have found impossible.

Just when Lois thought their life had stabilized, Pat suffered a back injury at work, underwent major surgery to fuse vertebrae, and was homebound, drawing a meager workman's compensation check. For the next eighteen months, Lois struggled to meet their financial needs by cleaning houses, low-paid, demanding work that she stoically accepted. Now prayer became even more important to her, especially when she thought wistfully of the freedom a divorce would bring. One of her counselors, an emotionally mature member of their church, offered Lois a "life scripture" from Psalm 37: "Trust in the Lord, and do good; Dwell in the land and cultivate faithfulness." To Lois this became a calming anchor, a personal assurance that the long struggle of her marriage was a battle worth waging.

During this period, members of King's Park International Church came forward with concrete aid. On the day when a major overdue payment would have provoked action from a collection service, the church secretary called Lois. An anonymous member had left an envelope with a thousand dollars in cash for them. All told, church members contributed more than three thousand dollars during the most desperate weeks of this crisis.

"If that's not a miracle," Lois told Pat, "I don't know what is."

As with other struggling couples, it would be gratifying if I could report that all of Pat and Lois's problems have been so miraculously resolved. But they have not. Although he has shown incredible strength and has also remained a kind and thoughtful person throughout this hardship, Pat must continue to struggle with his neurological condition. The couple's second daughter, Sarah, has a serious congenital illness that will require lifetime care. Yet Pat and Lois have matured as a couple, and now enjoy a warm and stable marriage that many less religious and more affluent people would do well to emulate. I can confidently restate the obvious: Without the emotional sustenance of strong religious faith and spiritual practices such as prayer and devotional reading, Pat and Lois's marriage would have been ripped apart by the stress of the multiple problems they have confronted. But I am amazed at how cheerful and optimistic they both have remained.

There are people who would argue that Lois, an educated and energetic woman, has wasted her best years trying to overcome seemingly endless problems. And, without doubt, many less religious women would have sought divorce when there appeared to be no relief from the nagging stress. For Lois this was never a viable option. Her basic love for Pat was strained, but not broken, during their long ordeal. Her faith had taught Lois that God tests each of us according to a plan we can never grasp with our limited human understanding. Therefore, she reasoned, it would have been an arrogant mistake to give in to her own "selfish" needs and limited sight by ending the marriage.

Surviving Hardships

I have found compelling research to account for the happiness and satisfaction Lois receives from her marriage, despite the serious hardships she and Pat have confronted. In the mid-1980s, researchers Margaret Wilson and Eric Filsinger studied 190 white married couples from a southwestern city, and found a high level of marital satisfaction among people who derived positive emotional reinforcement from traditional religious experiences. Certainly, Lois and Pat Cox's reliance on prayer, devotional reading, and group worship at church fits this definition of religious practice. There is mounting research evidence to support Wilson and Filsinger's conclusion that "higher religiosity predicts marital adjustment."[13]

Deriving strength from their faith to surmount marital problems is not unique to evangelical Protestants. Other researchers have found evidence that the level of church attendance among Roman Catholics accurately predicted happiness in marriage. This appears to be especially true among Catholics who marry within the faith and frequently attend mass together.[14] Further, studies have found a similar connection between strong faith and satisfaction in marriage among Seventh-Day Adventists in the Midwest.[15]

Lois Cox's attitude toward her marriage might be considered backward and wrongheaded in today's often hedonistic cultural milieu. But there is mounting scientific evidence that religion plays an important role in preventing divorce. In 1994, for example, Portland State University researcher Howard Weinberg studied the factors influencing the attempted marital reconciliations of 506 women selected from a nationwide sociological survey. Weinberg found that:

Religion appears to have an important impact on the success of a reconciliation. In particular, women having the same religion as their spouse have a significantly increased probability of having a successful reconciliation. Religious compatibility may affect the success of a reconciliation in that religion plays a role in everyday life such as the rearing and educating of children, the choice of where to live and who to socialize with, and the allocation of time and resources. The traditions, values, and sense of community that the couple share by having the same religion may act to help keep the reconciliation intact.[16]

In view of such evidence, and as a psychiatrist who regularly works with deeply dissatisfied people, I consider Pat and Lois's ongoing struggle a testimony to the healing power of faith.

Living in the Shadow of Danger: Mary and Glenn's Story

Military families can face severe stress unique to their demanding circumstances. Long separations, substandard housing, frequent moves that disrupt schooling, and repeated tours of hazardous duty are common challenges to members of the military, their spouses, and their children. Many military marriages cannot hold up under this chronic strain. But a surprising number of married couples thrive under the demands of military life. A deep, shared religious faith is often a significant factor preserving these families.

Mary and Glenn Nordin of San Antonio recently celebrated their forty-second wedding anniversary in the company of their four children and a growing throng of grandchildren.

Slender and animated, Mary appears much younger than her late sixties. Her husband Glenn, sixty-nine, is wiry and youthful. He speaks in a quiet, almost scholarly manner. But Glenn spent most of his adult life as an air force fighter-pilot and survived some of the most savage aerial combat of the Vietnam War.

The Nordins married in Michigan right out of college, where Glenn received a ROTC commission as an air force lieutenant. Although he had been raised in a conventional Lutheran home, it was Mary who brought a deeply personal religious faith to the marriage.

Their first years together would have strained any couple. Glenn was assigned the risky, thankless duty of ferrying single-engine jet fighters around the world, which always involved transoceanic flights relying on primitive navigational instruments to find vital refueling stops on islands. As Mary and Glenn's family grew, he was often away from home. Mary was constantly aware of the danger Glenn faced as she'd see the dreaded blue air force sedan carrying the chaplain to console yet another wife whose husband's plane had flown into a cloud-covered mountainside in the Mediterranean or disappeared into the blue void of the Pacific. Daily prayer and Bible reading sustained her.

For Glenn, who loved flying almost as much as he did his family, prayer assumed an important place in his regular "checklist" of activities. His religious faith helped Glenn accept the continual risks of his profession. Whenever he had a close encounter with death, he reminded himself that Mary was a strong moral person who would have the fortitude to raise their four children well, even in his absence.

In 1967 and 1968 Glenn was an F-4 Phantom pilot flying combat missions in Vietnam. His tour of duty coincided with an intense aerial campaign against enemy supply lines in North Vietnam and along the Ho Chi Minh Trail. Glenn's unit suffered high casualties, with a number of his colleagues killed, captured, or missing. Mary waited in America for him to return, shouldering the full responsibility of raising their four young children. In December 1967, Glenn's plane was hit by enemy fire as he prepared to land at the Da Nang air base. Glenn and his crewmate managed to eject a fractured second before the fighter exploded in a fireball. But when they landed by parachute in the mangrove swamp below, they were surrounded by the Vietcong unit that had shot down their plane. Miraculously, an American helicopter arrived overhead, and the two men struggled aboard the chopper as enemy bullets cracked around them.

Hours later in America, Mary received a shocking and confused message: Glenn's plane had been shot down, but he was apparently safe. As was her habit, she gathered her children around her and prayed intensely. She was calm when word finally reached her that Glenn was in fact uninjured.

Today, in their retirement, faith still plays an important role in the Nordins' personal life and marriage. Their four children are all religious, and several are leaders in their church congregation.

Reflecting on the important role faith played in their eventful and risk-filled life together, Mary Nordin notes simply, "I was taught that God brings strength to a family."

There is increasing evidence that Mary Nordin's traditional view of religion and family life is valid. Researcher Linda Robinson found strong confirmation that a couple's religious faith influences the stability and happiness of their marriage through moral guidance and social, emotional, and spiritual support. Religious faith seems to enhance other positive qualities that increase the happiness and satisfaction of married couples, "particularly intimacy, commitment, and communication." Robinson's study suggests that faith helps both individual spouses and couples in their marriages.[17]

Bringing Religious Marital Counseling Home

The most successful religious marital counseling efforts stress the equal partnership of husband and wife.

A good example of such an endeavor is the expanding Retrouvaille organization sponsored by the Roman Catholic church in many countries around the world. Retrouvaille ("Rediscovery") began in Canada in 1977 and emphasizes honest self-appraisal and better communication among couples. Known as a "lifeline for troubled marriages," the program starts with a Retrouvaille Weekend intended to help married people learn to listen, forgive, and speak to each other more openly. Couples who have saved their marriages, led by a priest coordinator, relate their experiences of overcoming disillusionment and angry conflict. Although the weekend is not a spiritual retreat, many participants draw on religious faith to overcome the pain connected with emotional healing and maturation.

In the three months following the first weekend, Retrouvaille clients are encouraged to participate in twelve presentations that focus on fundamental aspects of married life, including religious faith, forgiveness, and the sanctity of marriage. Mary Alice Breilinger, of the Family Life Apostolate of the Archdiocese of Boston, notes that Retrouvaille has a very high marital reconciliation rate when compared with purely secular counseling. Although the program is endorsed by the Catholic Church, it is open to all married couples, regardless of their religion. Readers can learn more about Retrouvaille by calling, toll-free, 1-800-470-2230, or contacting the group's Internet home page: www.retrouvaille.org/home.htm. Any inquiries can be kept strictly confidential.

One couple, whose marriage was saved by the program, frankly commented, "Retrouvaille hasn't eliminated our problems, but has given us the tools to work with. We have a better understanding of each other and the maturity to work things out instead of fighting." I can't think of a better endorsement for any effort meant to strengthen the bond joining a married couple.

The continuing high divorce rate proves that many couples lack the emotional strength needed to dig in and work toward building a strong family in today's world. I don't have to remind readers that the pressures and temptations of everyday life combine into a virtual centrifuge that is tearing marriages apart at an alarming pace. Couples can learn more about pastoral marriage counseling from a priest, minister, or rabbi simply by calling or visiting places of worship in their communities.

Recently, the State of Louisiana officially recognized that the type of commitment found in traditional religiously based marriages could provide a strong foundation for successful families. The state legislature passed the Covenant Marriage Act in 1997. A couple contracting a Covenant Marriage in Louisiana legally agree to several apparently archaic requirements. They must sign a declaration of intent acknowledging that their marriage is an institution that can be dissolved only under certain rigorous conditions.

＊

First, the couple must obtain premarital counseling from a "priest, minister, rabbi, or similar clergyman of any religious sect, or a marriage counselor."[18] The only legal grounds for separation or divorce in a Louisiana Covenant Marriage are adultery, the long imprisonment of the other spouse, abandonment, physical or sexual abuse in the family, or a period of separation of at least two years. Several other states have similar legislation pending in their legislatures.

I believe this Louisiana law formally recognizes what I have long observed: Religious faith often provides a solid foundation for strong marriages and families.

Chapter Four

✳

Religious People Have Healthy Lifestyles

I am sure you'll agree that the world's major religions encourage healthy living. Some even mandate abstention or moderation as basic dogma. Devout Hindus are strict vegetarians, as are many traditional Buddhists. The dietary laws of Judaism, kashruth, date from the earliest books of the Bible. Few pious Muslims drink alcohol.[1] Mormons and Seventh-Day Adventists practice healthy temperance in their daily lives. All established religions discourage drunkenness, risky sexual behavior, and any habit or activity harmful to the human body, which has traditionally been viewed as sacred, created in the image of God.

A growing array of research is charting the benefits to physical health that religious people often enjoy. I'm particularly impressed by studies showing that adolescents from strong religious backgrounds who frequently attend worship service, pray, and read scripture are far less likely to drink alcohol, smoke tobacco, or experiment with illegal drugs than their nonreligious peers.[2] Research also indicates premarital sexual intercourse is far less common among religious adolescents than among less religious teenagers.[3]

And there's convincing evidence that the shield of religious moderation continues into adulthood.[4] These lifestyle attitudes are the basis of the much lower rates of alcohol- and tobacco-related afflictions and sexually transmitted diseases among the religious when compared with their secular peers.

A Health-Promoting Network

I have also found that membership in a congregation can bring people other, less obvious health advantages. As we've seen with Walter and Marguerite Grounds and Khalita Jones, a congregation can become a person's second family. There is often sincere mutual love, concern, and respect among members of a faith community.[5] This social bond can become an informal health-promotion network. If a normally observant person begins to miss worship service, friends will call or visit. This can translate into a higher level of disease detection among members. In addition, a growing number of churches and synagogues have congregational health programs, which formalize this practice and also provide regular screening for heart disease, high blood pressure, many common cancers, and diabetes. My experience in family and geriatric medicine has taught me that screening and early illness detection are a vital part of wellness that people too often ignore. Many faith communities also sponsor groups to help members break dependence on drugs or alcohol, follow healthier eating habits, or control their weight.

In fact, congregational support groups and substance abuse programs are becoming so popular that they fell target to satirical cartoonist Garry Trudeau's "Doonesbury," where Baby Boomer pastor Scott Sloan's trendy church seemed to provide all his flock's needs, except, of course, traditional weekly worship. Despite Trudeau's good-natured ribbing, I am continually impressed with the power of faith-based recovery from drug or alcohol abuse. As I discovered with Lee Daugherty's unlikely rescue from terminal alcoholism in San Francisco, faith can provide the strength to break life-threatening addictions against which conventional interventions have proven powerless.

Overcoming Addiction: Rick's Story

I believe that the story of a man I will call Rick gives a human face to the growing body of scientific evidence that religion can help deliver seemingly hopeless drug addicts from a degrading life, or pointless death, on our cities' streets.[6]

Rick grew up during the 1950s in a stable African-American home in North Philadelphia. Both his parents worked well-paid factory jobs. They made a token effort to send their children to church on Sundays, but were not themselves members of a church. Rick's only brush with the law came when local beat cops caught him and his teenage pals with a pilfered bottle of wine.

He graduated from high school with good grades and hoped to study fashion design. But those dreams were sidetracked when his girlfriend announced she was pregnant. Five years later, Rick was the father of two little girls, completing an ironworker's union apprenticeship during the construction boom of the late 1970s.

"Those fat paychecks were a temptation," Rick now admits. He began "hanging out" at weekend parties with old friends. His wife complained, but Rick argued that he worked hard all week and deserved a little fun. After experimenting with marijuana, Rick moved on to methamphetamine. One night at a party Rick spread the pinch of white powder heroin on the back of his hand as instructed, held his fist to his nose, and snorted deeply. The sensual rush was overpowering, like sexual pleasure that seemed to last for hours.

Within three months, Rick was addicted. Work meant nothing; his wife and children became nagging strangers bent on depriving him of pleasure. He lost his job, bled his family's savings, and turned his back on everyone who tried to keep him from heroin. His family left the week the bank repossessed their house, and he and his wife subsequently divorced. Buddies from work, his family, and even retired cops from the old neighborhood begged Rick to seek treatment. "I can take it or leave it alone," he said, the classic words of an addict's denial.

A year later, scared by his now undeniable addiction, Rick voluntarily joined a city treatment program. But he dropped out when a guy from the street slipped him a small bag of heroin.

The next summer, his ex-wife and his parents finally persuaded him to undergo detoxification at an established private hospital, a combination of tranquilizer therapy and intense counseling, lasting weeks.

"Your body is free of opiates, Rick," doctors eventually assured him. In counseling, Rick voiced his sincere desire to break the addiction. "I really do want to live a clean life."

But there had not been one conscious moment during those weeks when Rick had not been painfully aware of the burning tingle in his belly, reminding him of the sensual glow that just one little bag of heroin could deliver.

Rick completed the program on a hot August afternoon in 1990. Less than three hours later, he was in his car, cruising the streets of North Philadelphia, searching for a heroin fix. Throughout his treatment, no matter the words he spoke or heard, a wakeful, silent corner of his mind focused on one immutable image: a plastic bag hardly bigger than a postage stamp bulging with snowy powder heroin.

Experts on addiction have discovered that especially stubborn addicts such as Rick might truly wish to kick drugs on the conscious level, but that more basic centers of their brains are deaf to all words of counsel and guidance. Those millions of unseen cells, their microscopic receptors virtually quivering for the next opiate rush, care nothing for good intentions.

Rick was soon living on the streets, a junkie dealer in an expendable stable run by a drug gang. Rick worked for dope, earning the right to keep one bag out of every ten-bag bundle he sold. Days passed without eating, malt liquor his only fluid. Some nights he would wake, craving a fix, on the floor of a foul shooting gallery where addicts rented syringes. The months, even the seasons, became a blur in Rick's mind. But certain images were so terrible that they burned through the heroin veil.

One windy fall night, he worked the streets among gaunt teenage prostitutes. A flurry of color caught his interest. One of the girls clutched the hand of a toddler decked out in a bright slicker emblazoned with a *Sesame Street* Muppet. The girl handed the child to one of her "sisters," then climbed into the car of a suburban customer. Rick pictured his own little daughters, a vision so painful that he ripped open an unsold bundle of heroin and snorted a bag right on the street.

During a harsh spring ice storm, Rick haunted his usual corners, angry at the lack of customers. Then he saw two boys in gaudy Starter jackets clomping toward him through the slush. He realized too late they were the predators who had already shot down two street dealers for their drug stashes earlier that winter. The smaller boy dragged a huge pistol from his jacket and pointed it at Rick, his hands shaking beneath the weight. Rick ran, his heart thudding in panic, then slipped and twisted his knee. When he finally limped into the sanctuary of his dealer's shooting gallery, Rick was trembling. "How old *is* that kid with the big gun?" he asked. " 'Bout ten, I reckon," the dealer replied.

Over the next two years, Rick was arrested four times. But he jumped bond, skipped trials, and began living as a fugitive, holed up at night on a stinking mattress in an abandoned factory. At dawn one freezing winter morning, he woke to the thud of gunfire just outside. A young man screamed, begging for help. A car drove off; the young man whimpered like a wounded animal. Rick rolled over and snorted the half bag of heroin he'd been saving. "He's better off dead," Rick whispered, then sat upright, the drug useless against the chill image that gripped him. "I'm going to die alone just like that poor kid outside."

But ten days later, he met one of his dealer friends on a busy corner. The man looked healthy; there was a bounce to his step. "Hey, man," Rick said. "You score somethin' big?"

His friend smiled. "I'm clean, bro." He grinned. "You can be too. It ain't hard."

Rick shook his head. He felt no desire to stand in line at yet another methadone clinic. "It ain't no 'M-down,' " his friend reassured him.

He led Rick to an evangelical shelter called "The Way to Heaven." The echoing dormitory seemed bare. But the beds were clean, the showers hot, the food nourishing. Rick had not slept on clean sheets for two years. When he woke, he warily joined a prayer circle of men like himself, both African-American and Hispanic, seated in a ring, clutching each other's hands for strength. A pastor named Rosado read from the Bible, assuring the men that the gospel applied to them. Rick closed his eyes against the loud voice. *No way Jesus going to love a strung-out junkie like me.*

As if reading his thoughts, a counselor named George Ortiz gripped

Rick's shoulder. Ortiz held his Bible open to Hebrews 13:5. "Rick," Ortiz said confidently, "Jesus told everyone who believed, 'I will never leave you nor forsake you.' He meant people like me and *you*."

Rick seized the book and leaned close to study the words. "Say it out loud," Ortiz urged.

Rick began to repeat the passage, a personal liturgy he intoned for hours that day, into the night, and on toward the rainy dawn, when the hungry fire in his belly flared hottest. He lay on his bunk, rocking in a fetal position, the Bible pressed to his face, speaking the words until sleep finally overtook him. An image of a strong but infinitely gentle pair of hands protecting his body as Rick had once shielded a chirping baby sparrow in his parents' backyard slowly grew in his mind. The craving for heroin had somehow slipped outside beyond this shield. " 'I will never leave you. . . .' "

It was a warm Indian summer Wednesday night when George Ortiz took Rick to the huge Deliverance Evangelistic Church on Twenty-first Street and Lehigh Avenue. Rick flushed with embarrassment as George led him down the gleaming tile hallway to the weekly Drug Task Force session. *Man*, he thought, *these people really don't want someone like me in a nice church like this.* But he fell back on his scriptural passage, "I will never leave you. . . ."

During the prayer and personal testimony that night, Rick felt an unexpected flow of comfort when he gripped hands with these nicely dressed, well-spoken men. How could they ever have been junkies like him? Yet their personal stories were every bit as squalid as his own. Some had been street dealers, others pimps; all knew the reality of drugs.

That Sunday, Rick joined the Deliverance congregation in the wide church amphitheater for the first time. The hundreds of cheerful black families reminded him of a childhood world he had feared was extinct. Then the pastor, Reverend Ben Smith, a husky man in his seventies with magnetic eyes and a strong, unquavering voice, called for the "lost sheep" to approach the altar. Rick was suddenly moving forward as if dragged by an unseen force. His right hand rose to show his commitment to God. As his arm reached full extension, he was flooded with a bright warmth even more intense than the euphoria of a heroin rush.

In the coming weeks, Rick learned how extensive the family that called Deliverance their spiritual home actually was. The congregation included a dozen specialized ministries and outreach programs. Deliverance's prison ministry trained volunteers to take the gospel to incarcerated men and women, many of whom had become law-abiding, taxpaying citizens. Volunteers from the home care department provided hot meals, housecleaning, and companionship to hundreds of shut-in elderly people across North Philadelphia. Rick met pastors from the youth program who nightly walked the streets of the city's toughest drug gang turfs, spreading the Word.

Rick's sponsors introduced him to church members trained in drug rehabilitation, criminal justice, and job counseling. His new spiritual family accompanied him to each court appearance that fall, insisting he "make good" on every outstanding warrant. The court granted Rick probation, provided he remain in drug counseling at Deliverance.

After the elation of that first Sunday, Rick faced the hard challenge known to all addicts in recovery: how to stay clean and not fall back on drugs during times of stress. Although Rick still drew comfort from his personal scriptural passage, his counselors taught him a prayer to recite when he was most vulnerable: "Lord, help me to hate this drug as much as I once loved it." Rick repeated this prayer a hundred times a day. Initially skeptical that this seemingly simple invocation would quench the burning for heroin that had never cooled during all the psychotherapy and drug treatment he had undergone, Rick was soon convinced. He acquired an actual physical revulsion at the mere thought of heroin. For the first time in years, the churning heat in his belly had been extinguished.

A year later, Rick became partners in a home renovation business with his first drug counselor, George Ortiz. Rick married one of the church officers and has reconciled with his two children.

Recently, Rick's job took him to the neighborhood where he had once dealt heroin. He saw a bony specter of a young street dealer in a stained army jacket, hunched against a telephone pole. There had to be dope in those jacket pockets, little white bags of heroin nestled like sleeping eggs. In another life less than two years earlier, this vision would have sparked the fiery hunger in Rick's belly. But now he smiled with a serene calm.

"You high on somethin'?" the dealer asked.

"Yeah," Rick answered. "I guess I am. But it's nothing you can buy or sell." He gave the man a card from the Deliverance Drug Task Force, gripped his shoulder, and urged him to come to the next Wednesday night meeting.

Religion, Mood, and Neurotransmitters

Is Rick's recovery an intriguing fluke, irrelevant to the plights of the more than one million addicts haunting our streets? There is increasing scientific evidence to the contrary. One of the pioneering studies on the power of religious faith to heal addicts' longing for heroin was funded by the National Institute on Drug Abuse in the late 1970s.[7] David P. Desmond, at the University of Texas Health Science Center in San Antonio, led research on male heroin addicts undergoing treatment at a local Public Health Service hospital, some of whom later joined inpatient religious recovery programs. A year into recovery, those in the religious-based recovery programs were almost eight times more likely to report abstinence from opiates than those who received purely secular treatment.[8]

From the pure perspective of medical science, addicted people who turn to religion to change their lives probably derive both emotional *and* physiological support from the practice of their faith. Again, we have persuasive evidence that deeply sincere devotional practices—Rick's healing reliance on the verse from Hebrews, Lee Daugherty's daily recitations from the Book of Psalms—reduce stress. In other words, people worshiping in this manner enjoy improved mood; they are delivered from anguished tension to tranquillity. And we know mood is connected to chemical neurotransmitters in our brains, such as serotonin. Neuroscientists now believe many people suffering from depression have low levels of certain neurotransmitters, which seems to predispose them to drug or alcohol abuse. "Drown your sorrows" might be a shopworn adage, but it is an accurate metaphor for many substance abusers' effort to ease their emotional pain. We don't yet know, however, if depression is the cause or the effect of chemical imbalance in the brain.

But we have evidence that addicts undergoing religious recovery do not *feel* the intense craving for drugs that once ruled their lives. It seems reasonable to expect, therefore, that future research would explore the possibility that individual and group prayer, song worship, and devotional reading might affect the same centers of the brain that are stimulated by anxiety-reducing drugs such as opiates, alcohol, and cocaine. The scientific jury is a long way from reaching its final verdict on this point. We do know, however, as Rick's story illustrates, that the intensity of profound religious emotions can at least ease the inner turmoil of many drug addicts.

"High" on Religion

Certainly intense spiritual events can produce monumental and seemingly inexplicable changes in a person's life. Consider Paul the Apostle's blinding conversion on the road to Damascus. (At the time he was a rabbinically trained Pharisee named Saul of Tarsus, so proud of his Roman citizenship that he adopted the latinized name Paulus.) In one moment, he was transformed into the Roman world's strongest advocate of the gospel of Jesus of Nazareth. In this century, mass revival meetings have evoked similar strong responses in millions of people. And Rick felt an immense flood of healing grace when he answered the altar call and raised his hand to publicly acknowledge his need for salvation before the huge, supportive Deliverance congregation. How much do we know about what actually happens physically in people's brains at such moments? Not very much.

Perhaps addiction experts might now want to investigate possible similarities between the powerful "high" produced by drugs and the intense religious joy felt by former addicts such as Rick who have recovered through an emotionally intense conversion experience.

One interesting study from the 1980s examined young adult psychiatric patients being treated for what we call "affective disorders," including psychotic depression, mania, and bipolar conditions, at university medical centers in the East and Midwest. These conditions are primarily biological disorders that we think are due to imbalances in brain chemistry. People suffering these disorders often try to ease their emotional pain with illicit drugs or alcohol (in a behavior called "self-medication"). But the researchers found significantly lower rates of drug and alcohol abuse among the patients who were highly involved with their religious faith.[9] This might indicate that satisfying religious experience offers a healthy inner peace to people at risk for depression who otherwise might seek comfort in drugs or alcohol.

Is Religion Just Another Addiction?

I have heard people cynically comment that a person addicted to drugs merely "trades one addiction for another" by embracing religion. I strongly reject this view. As a physician, one of my principal responsibilities is to alleviate human suffering and work toward improving people's quality of life. But frankly, there are conditions, including some cases of addiction to alcohol or drugs, against which medicine has proven largely powerless. Obviously, Rick's quality of life improved after his religious conversion gave him the strength to abandon drugs. And I hope that rational people would concur that a healthy religious life is preferable to the slow death of addiction that Rick faced.

Helping Each Other: Monty's Story

One of the most compelling aspects of Rick's recovery is the dedication of many former addicts, healed through religion, to help those still in the grip of drugs or alcohol.

By the fall of 1984, Monty Cox, then forty-three, had reached that terrible place alcoholics call "the pit." He lived in an abandoned house with no running water, heat, or electricity on a sprawling hog farm along the tidewater flats of lower Delaware. At almost six feet and less than 130 pounds, Monty had become a teetering skeletal husk. In this terminal stage of his addiction he drank almost a quart of cheap whiskey a day, sipping during "working" hours and guzzling the remaining half bottle until he passed out each night. When he remembered to eat, food was a can of tuna and a few crackers. There had once been a wife and children living here with him in this hovel. They had disappeared, so he forgot about them.

His job was suited to his condition. Each week he had to muck out the three large hog houses with a pressure hose. But Monty's brain was so fogged by alcohol that he could not remember the correct weekly cleaning sequence. So, three times a week, his boss carefully printed a note of exact orders and stuck it in Monty's shirt pocket. "House three today, Monty," he would shout, as if speaking to a retarded person.

One chill November morning the owner found Monty lying rigid with terror on his dingy mattress. "The *rats*," Monty hissed, waving his skinny hand at the peeling wallpaper. "Rats everywhere." But the rats only existed in his delirium tremens hallucinations. The man drove Monty to the state detox unit in Ellendale, Delaware. That night a nurse mixed two ounces of grain alcohol into a glass of orange juice for him to drink. "You've been walking around for years with a three-point-five blood alcohol level," she noted with alarm. "It's going to take weeks to bring you down safely."

But when Monty woke in the clinic the next morning, his head was clear, and he could remember people and events he had not thought of for years. Monty reflected on almost twenty-four years of drinking that had begun with his first job as a sign painter in suburban Washington, D.C. In those years he had acquired and lost a family, passed through dozens of jobs, including high-pay work as an auto-body mechanic, but had always refused to surrender his precious whiskey bottle. On any normal morning, he would have groped beneath his mattress for his emergency pint and taken the first calming sips.

But lying here in this clean bed, geese honking in the sunny sky and yellow leaves falling in the breeze, Monty felt a languid calm he had not known since childhood. It was like Saturday morning with no school. *I don't want a drink,* he realized, stunned by the insight.

He rose cautiously, but found that his limbs were not shaking. He walked to a chair and stared out at the leaf-strewn lawn. Still the thirst was not snapping like a mousetrap beneath his throat. *Why?* Now Monty smelled the aroma of sausage and eggs from the kitchen. His stomach rumbled with hunger, not nausea. What was happening to him?

Facing the mirror above the lavatory sink, he saw a new glow in his eyes. Sudden insight washed over him like a powerful wave. "God wants me to be sober," he whispered, stunned by the revelation.

In the past, Monty Cox had scorned "Bible-pounding" do-gooders preaching sobriety. He had not attended church for decades, never read scripture. But the bizarre realization that God would provide him the strength to abandon alcohol was more real to him than anything he could remember.

After eating a big breakfast, he told the nurse he did not need his midday maintenance drink of alcohol and orange juice. She looked at him skeptically. "Come around when you do need it" was all she said.

But to the amazement of the medical staff, Monty Cox remained alcohol-free at the detox center. Then he entered the Willis Hudson Center for residential recovery in nearby Salisbury, Maryland. Monty's first day passed well, with his craving still extinguished. But the radio was tuned to a country-and-western station, music Monty associated with the smoky clapboard bars along Route 13. He could picture himself propped against the bar on payday, a fresh bottle of Club 400 whiskey and a double shot glass sitting by his elbow. The sleeping creature under his chest was beginning to wake. On an impulse, Monty changed the station. The dial swung to a local Christian program, *Joy!* A voice was speaking calmly about God's patience with sinners teetering on the brink of destruction. Monty sat on a bunk the rest of the afternoon, his face close to the radio.

That night, Monty was still absorbed in the prayer and devotional music when a patient offered to share a smuggled pint of whiskey.

*

Monty gazed at the brown bottle and the ornate label. He could see the amber liquid swirling inside. The thirst was still washing beneath his chest, almost mirroring the whiskey in the bottle. But he now knew firmly that God had another purpose in his life. "You ought to just flush that down the toilet," he gently told the man.

Monty lived for the next two years at the Christian Shelter, where he was befriended by a volunteer pastor, "Brother Russ" Ogden. When Monty described his almost painless physical withdrawal from alcohol addiction, Brother Russ smiled. "God did send you grace," he said. "Now you have to learn how to use it." The two men spent months in scriptural studies. Brother Russ urged Monty to read the beatitudes as a personal commandment to "Be these attitudes." Slowly, but with increasing conviction, Monty Cox absorbed the firm understanding that God had intervened directly in his life to save him from slow suicide by whiskey.

He decided to trust completely in divine will, which he was sure would lead him on the right path. After working as an unlicensed, shade-tree street mechanic for several months, Monty used his savings and a small loan to open his own business, the Chevette Shop. There were hundreds of these aging little GM econoboxes still on the road, owned mostly by kids, farmworkers, and families working as shuckers at the oyster houses. Monty would repair the old cars when the big dealers refused to do so. Chevette owners sought him out from surrounding states. Monty worked six days a week, ate well, prayed, read scripture, and didn't even think about the lovely brown curves of a Club 400 whiskey bottle.

When it came time to hire mechanics, Monty went back to the Christian Shelter. "I've got honest work for men wanting to start over."

In the last thirteen years, Monty Cox has hired scores of recovering alcoholics, prisoners on work release from the nearby Poplar Hill facility, and several young deaf men from a local state training school. Usually they stay with him long enough to get back on their feet, learn advanced skills, and then move on to better-paying jobs at big dealers. That's what Monty wants. He sees himself as a Christian decompression chamber, where men can pass from a life of degradation to a life of grace. His own life has definitely been graced. Monty has remarried. His wife, Leona, is a quietly religious person who shares Monty's gentle approach to working with recovering drug addicts and alcoholics. Leona does not object to the hours Monty spends each week working as a volunteer at the Willis Hudson Center or speaking at schools and churches about recovery. In an act of mercy that would have tried the most devout, Monty and Leona took in his mother and stepfather when they returned to Maryland from California, broke and dispirited. Monty's stepfather, a lifelong alcoholic, had suffered irreparable brain damage from decades of drinking. His memory and cognition had eroded to a level resembling advanced Alzheimer's disease. Even though Monty and Leona wanted to save for their own future retirement, they cheerfully spent five hundred dollars a week for the round-the-clock nursing care his stepfather required.

"I was almost walking in his shoes," Monty notes. "But by God's grace, I got my mind back."

Grace is a subject Monty discusses with all the men who pass through his workshop. On a recent rainy winter afternoon, Monty Cox spoke with quiet determination over the whine of grinders and the thump of fender tools, explaining the subtle differences between grace and gratitude to one of his new workers.

"Grace is a gift from God," Monty stated as if discussing some indisputable fact, perhaps the thickness of standard-gauge metal plate. Then, as he smiled broadly, his words became more animated. "Now, gratitude . . . that's taking God's gift and giving it to your fellow man."

The new worker, only ten days out of the Hudson Center and still amazed by sobriety, set down the can of body putty and repeated Monty Cox's healing words.

Studying Alcoholism and Religious Faith

Harvard Medical School psychiatrist and substance abuse pioneer George E. Valliant discussed the power of religion to heal drug and alcohol addiction in his classic book *The Natural History of Alcoholism: Causes, Patterns, and Paths to Recovery.*[10] Karl Marx's adage that religion is the "opiate of the masses," Valliant argues, masks the "enormously important therapeutic principle" of religious faith. To successfully recover from addiction, chronic drug and alcohol abusers need "powerful new sources of self-esteem and hope." Isn't that exactly what the Deliverance Drug Task Force provided Rick and what Brother Russ taught Monty Cox?

Dr. Valliant also offers an insight that I believe lies at the heart of faith's healing power over drugs and alcohol: "Religion provides fresh impetus for both hope and enhanced self-care." For alcoholics to achieve stable recovery, Valliant adds, they most undergo "enormous personality changes."

"It is not just coincidence," Valliant goes on, "that we associate such dramatic change with the experience of religious conversion." Again, try to imagine people such as Lee Daugherty or Monty Cox struggling against their addiction *without* the comforting strength of prayer or scripture.

Further, Valliant identifies forgiveness as a key factor in breaking the alcoholic's endless cycle of guilt and binging, followed by increased guilt, seeking relief in alcohol, and so on. For people like Lee Daugherty and Monty Cox, Valliant notes, "absolution becomes an important part of the healing process."[11] This was the intangible gift of grace that provided Rick and Monty the inner peace to turn away from addiction.

Most psychiatrists recognize that the oldest and most successful recovery organization, and the model for all "Twelve Step" programs, Alcoholics Anonymous, depends heavily on God and divine grace to achieve and preserve sobriety. AA members recite the Twelve Steps at each meeting; in Step Eleven they publicly concede that they have sought "through prayer and meditation to improve our conscious contact with God *as we understand Him,* praying only for knowledge of His will for us and the power to carry that out."[12]

*

Learning More: The Piedmont Study

To me, Monty Cox's reliance on divine grace to stay sober for more than fourteen years is a testimony to the power of religious faith to heal one of the most intractable addictions medicine faces. In 1994, I led a team of colleagues at Duke University on a detailed study of the relationship between religious practices and alcoholism among a large sampling of adult southerners whose faith, scriptural interest, and worship patterns appear similar to those of Monty Cox. The results of this study provide additional strong evidence that religion can help protect people from ravaging addiction to alcohol.[13]

We investigated almost three thousand adults from the Piedmont area of North Carolina, aged eighteen to ninety-seven, who had participated in the National Institute of Mental Health Epidemiologic Catchment Area survey in 1983–84. My team was testing several hypotheses on the possible benefits of religious faith and worship practices as a shield against alcohol abuse. Because our sample cut across age, race, and socioeconomic lines, we have confidence in the validity of our findings. Our basic yardstick was previous six-month and lifetime rates of alcohol abuse or dependence, as measured in the standard psychiatric manner (Third Edition of the *Diagnostic and Statistical Manual* [DSM-III]).

We used several questions to assess our subjects' religious faith and practices, focusing on: worship service attendance, private prayer, scriptural reading, personal importance of religion, and self-identification as a "born-again" Christian.

The survey was broad enough that we could question a large variety of conservative and mainline Protestants, Pentecostals, Catholics, and Eastern Orthodox, as well as a much smaller sampling of Jews, Jehovah's Witnesses, Mormons, and Unitarians.

Our results were quite provocative, and did not always follow our hypotheses. We found that:

- Recent alcohol abuse or dependence (in the six months preceding the survey) was significantly lower among people who frequently engaged in private worship, including prayer and scriptural study.

• Both recent and lifetime alcohol problems were lower among those who attended worship service.

• People who attended church at least weekly had less than one-third the rate of alcohol abuse of those who went less frequently.

• The reported personal importance of religion to people did not seem to be related to their risk of having alcohol problems.

• Religion may be a buffer against the onset of alcoholism, or help people achieve sobriety once addiction has set in.

We thought that people who described themselves as being born again would have low recent rates of alcohol abuse, but possibly have a background of alcoholism. In fact, both recent and lifetime rates of alcohol disorders were lower among born-again Christians than among others in the survey.

Another of our hypotheses was that overall risk of alcohol disorders would be lower among people from more conservative or fundamentalist denominations, which strongly discourage drinking. But we found no significant relationship between religious affiliation and recent alcohol abuse. On the other hand, lifetime rates of alcoholism were highest among Pentecostal Christians (17.4 percent of those questioned) and lowest among mainline and conservative Protestants (8.6 percent and 8.8 percent, respectively).

We considered it possible that some Pentecostals might be driven toward alcoholism by their denomination's "harsh and restrictive doctrines" toward alcohol. However, it seems more likely that Pentecostal Christianity's total rejection of alcohol, but not of the alcoholic, might provide comfort to addicted people, and therefore attract more of them. Further, our study noted, "Pentecostal groups emphasize positive emotional experience, which alcoholics typically seek." And finally, we found that Pentecostal churches welcome poorer people, whom mainstream congregations often discourage, and victims of emotional illness and alcoholism.[14]

Further research building on our study might one day demonstrate more clearly that people vulnerable to drug and alcohol addiction are attracted to the charismatic, emotionally satisfying experience of Pentecostal worship.[15]

Those in our study who reported regular private prayer and Bible reading had significantly lower rates of recent alcohol abuse. We believe our study provides evidence that private religious activities may protect people from alcohol disorders.

In general, all the apparent protective factors of religion were strongest among the adults aged eighteen to thirty-nine, and weakest among middle-age and elderly adults. So my team concluded that private and group religious activity may shield people from alcohol problems, and that this effect is particularly significant in younger adults. The personal odysseys of Lee Daugherty and Monty Cox are heartening examples of this last finding.

Jews Abuse Alcohol Too: Ruth's Story

There are illogical myths associated with most religions or major denominations. Baptists are said to be straitlaced, Catholics prone to gambling, Muslims male chauvinists. And "everybody" knows that Jewish alcoholics are very rare.

Unfortunately, as Shakespeare reminds us in *The Merchant of Venice*, Jews are made of the same vulnerable flesh and spirit as the rest of humanity. Alcoholism can afflict a Jewish woman in the affluent suburbs just as readily as it can devastate a blue-collar Christian man like Monty Cox. And Judaism can provide the grace needed to heal an apparently intractable alcohol addiction in the same manner as evangelical Christianity.

A woman I'll simply call Ruth offers a fine example of the healing power of faith over destructive alcohol dependence.

Ruth, now in early middle age, was raised in a basically nonreligious home, although she and her brother did occasionally attend synagogue Sunday school and he was bar mitzvahed as a social rite of passage. "But our family ignored the rich spiritual traditions of religion," Ruth recalls.

"My parents especially looked down on the obvious outward trappings of Judaism—the bearded Hasidim with their long black coats and archaic hats, the Orthodox men who wore yarmulkes out in public."

Ruth's family was rightfully proud of the major contributions of Jewish culture to science, philosophy, and the arts. "But our souls were not nourished as well as our intellects."[16]

Ruth believes this lack of a spiritual grounding in childhood contributed to her "desperate search for satisfaction" in young adulthood, when she first began to crave alcohol and prescription tranquilizers. Still a teenager, she married a man who successfully hid his worsening alcoholism under a veneer of professional achievement. By age thirty, she was living in an expensive home, driving a luxury car, and jetting around the world on business trips with her husband while their young children were cared for by a nanny.

Her husband turned to destructive amounts of alcohol to cope with mounting business stress. Although Ruth couldn't quite match his drinking, she exacerbated her own alcoholism with a growing dependence on Valium and other tranquilizers she could persuade compliant doctors to prescribe. "We maintained a pretty functional facade," Ruth says. But away from the public, her husband attacked her in violent, drunken rampages. He once chased her around the suite of an expensive hotel while she defended herself with a kitchen knife, screaming back each of his obscene threats. When sober, each bitterly blamed the other for the empty core of their glittering life.

Friends and relatives refused to recognize the obvious; alcoholism, after all, was not a Jewish problem. Fifteen years into the marriage, however, her husband's addiction could no longer be denied. Because he was now continually drunk, he lost his business, and with it the money to support their protective facade. Ruth "woke up to the truth." She was an alcoholic.

Ruth "dove" into Alcoholics Anonymous with the same compulsion that had once fueled her addiction. The Twelve Step program served her well. But after three years of sobriety, divorced and living a normal life, she still felt an aching emotional void. Then she heard about a retreat for recovering alcoholics and other addicts offered by Jewish Alcoholics, Chemically Dependent Persons and Significant Others (JACS), an affiliate of the Jewish Board of Family and Children's Services in New York.

"I was amazed when I walked into that shabby old hotel in the Catskills," Ruth remembers. There were over two hundred Jewish men and women just like her, including distinguished rabbis and the Hasidim with the beards and long black coats she had disparaged in childhood. "They were definitely alcoholics," she says with an ironic smile. "And nobody could deny they were also Jews." Just being among so many Jewish people openly admitting their problem bolstered Ruth's confidence.

But that night when she attended a religious service in the old resort's ballroom, her spiritual recovery gathered momentum. Reading unfamiliar, transliterated Hebrew prayers, Ruth joined the unofficial congregation asking God to grace those addicts who had not yet recovered from their bondage. She sat beside a tall Hasidic man whose cutaway coat bunched up awkwardly on the folding chair. The soft-spoken man patiently taught her to pronounce the Hebrew text in the Torah. For the first time, she heard her own voice speaking sacred words that dated from the ancient tribal origins of the Jewish people. Chanting the prayers, Ruth had the distinct sensation that this was liturgy she had somehow known her entire life.

Later, as she sat in a corner of the ballroom, eyes closed, meditating with a rabbi, she felt a cooling presence sweep through her. "I guess that was an angel," Ruth says. That night she realized that divine grace had supported her during all the hellish, drunken years of her marriage, and that grace still protected her in her ongoing recovery.

Since that first gathering in the Catskills eleven years ago, Ruth has attended JACS retreats twice a year. Judaism has given her a spiritual foundation on which to rebuild her life. She keeps a kosher home with her new husband and always observes the Sabbath.

"My life is full and satisfying to an extent I would not have believed possible," Ruth said recently. Like most former alcoholics, Ruth sometimes struggles to maintain her recovery. During times of stress, she meditates on the psalms of King David, carefully pronouncing the elegant Hebrew of the ageless liturgy. "Every day has its own unexpected spiritual dimension that I would not have known without reconnecting to the religion of my soul."

Nicotine Addiction: The North Carolina Study

I think it's clear that drug abuse and alcoholism are serious threats to our nation's health. But tobacco is probably the single most injurious legal substance still in wide use today. In particular, cigarette smoking has been shown to increase the risk for developing cancer of the lung, mouth, and throat and several other dangerous malignancies, including leukemia and myeloma. Smoking is also a major factor in high blood pressure, fatal respiratory diseases, and overall premature death. In fact, smoking accounts for almost half of the difference in mortality rate between American men and women.[17] And a convincing body of research shows that nicotine addiction is among the most stubborn substance abuse problems we face.

But can religion protect people against the harmful effects of tobacco addiction? A large research study by our Duke research team found evidence that this may indeed be the case.[18] We compared the religious beliefs and practices of almost four thousand randomly selected older people living in North Carolina with their patterns of cigarette smoking. I should note that North Carolina is both the "buckle" of the Bible Belt and also the most solid bastion of the tobacco industry. Cigarette smoking has been prevalent here for decades, which makes the state the ideal setting for the study of the relationship between religion and smoking.

We chose our subjects from the National Institutes of Health–sponsored Establishment of Populations for Epidemiologic Studies of the Elderly (EPESE).

We measured people's religious activities by attendance at church services and frequency of prayer, meditation, scriptural study, and viewing religious television or listening to religious radio programs. We also took into consideration people's physical health. Our researchers determined a person's level of cigarette smoking (if any) by asking detailed questions about present and past smoking habits. This determined the number of "pack years" for the smokers. Finally, we tried to determine our subjects' alcohol habits.

The findings were highly significant:

• Older adults who frequently attended religious service or engaged in private prayer or Bible study were much less likely to smoke cigarettes, and if they did, smoked fewer cigarettes a day than their less religiously active peers.
• Analyzing subject groups in chronological "waves" (1986, 1989, 1992), we found private religious activity, such as individual prayer or Bible study, a good indication that people were likely to never smoke cigarettes.
• Our most important finding was that people who *both* attended religious services at least once a week and prayed or studied the Bible at least daily were almost 90 percent more likely not to smoke than people less involved in these religious activities.
• Being part of the large religious broadcast audience did not protect people from smoking. But those who smoked and also frequently watched or listened to religious programs consumed fewer cigarettes per day than other smokers.

Nearly 60 percent of our sample were Baptist, a conservative Protestant denomination that often teaches respect for one's physical body as the "temple of the Holy Spirit." This attitude might account for these people's moderate habits. Nevertheless, they came of age during the Great Depression and World War II, when smoking was an inexpensive and popular way to cope with widespread stress. I found it very interesting that the lower rates of cigarette smoking among these religiously active older people were not due to their having broken the habit, but rather to their *never having smoked*. That demonstrates a remarkable level of resistance to peer pressure for North Carolinians of their generation. Again, however, research has demonstrated lower levels of anxiety, alcohol abuse, and depression among religiously active people.

I don't know if we can generalize our findings about smoking and religion for the entire country. But for years Gallup polls have found that most older Americans tend to be quite religious. The leaders of the growing antismoking movement would do well to consider the evidence that religious faith might prevent people from smoking, assist them in quitting the habit, or help them smoke less if they have already begun.

Escaping the Drug Culture: Bruce and Jackie's Story

Many young people drift into the drug culture as a result of peer pressure. Is religious faith enough to help them break free? The lives of a Midwestern couple I will call Bruce and Jackie dramatize the power of religious faith to shield young people from the temptation of drug experimentation. Now approaching middle age, Bruce and Jackie survived a frightening odyssey through their drug culture in the 1970s largely thanks to their religious conversion.

Bruce grew up in a suburban home in a Midwestern industrial city, the second of five children. His father was a mid-level manager. The family lived in a comfortable split-level on a quiet cul-de-sac near a wooded creek bed, a seemingly ideal white middle-class neighborhood, far removed from the inner city's endemic crime and drugs that are paraded across the ten o'clock news each night. Jackie was raised in a similar middle-class family and suburb on the other side of town.

Bruce entered the large, modern suburban high school in the mid-1970s, Jackie arrived the next year. Neither had thought much about drugs before high school; certainly their parents hadn't been concerned about the problem. Marijuana and LSD seemed to be alien substances used by weird hippies in New York's East Village or the Haight-Ashbury district in San Francisco.

But the situation changed with terrifying speed. "I smoked my first joint in October of my freshman year," Bruce later recalled. By the next spring, he was using marijuana every weekend. That summer, he "tried a couple pills," including bootlegged tranquilizers and methamphetamines. He estimates that by his senior year a solid majority of the students were regularly using illicit drugs. That year Bruce had progressed to the point of regularly smoking a full joint each morning before school. Weekends became "heavy partying" binges of tranquilizers and alcohol, methamphetamine, and occasionally LSD.

When Bruce stumbled home, "stoned out of my gourd," his parents thought he'd been experimenting with beer, a normal teenage problem.

But that summer they found an array of drug paraphernalia, including syringes and laboratory scales, sloppily hidden in Bruce's room. Now the Good Housekeeping tranquillity of their home collapsed into bitter arguments. Bruce refused to admit he had a drug problem. He also refused to apply for college or get a job. In frustration, his father ordered him out of the house. Bruce left, screaming obscenities at his parents.

Jackie's battle with drugs paralleled Bruce's. By her third year at high school, she belonged to a loose group of "deadbeat" LSD users. "I dropped every kind of acid you could find," she remembers, "Mr. Natural, Sunshine, stuff that was supposed to be straight from the Sandoz lab." Jackie drifted into a dangerous "Harley rider" motorcycle gang that frequented convenience stores on her side of the city. She added quaalude "wall-bangers" to her regular LSD consumption. Her parents eventually issued an ultimatum: Give up dope or leave home. Jackie left.

Bruce followed a pal to the Sunbelt, where he heard there was high-paying work in the oil fields. Jackie joined him a few weeks later. They found themselves living in a rented trailer, working for minimum wage, rationing their dwindling supply of LSD and barbiturates. When the dope ran low, they switched to beer and whiskey. Drunkenness led to screaming fights.

One hungover Sunday morning, Jackie suggested they might try visiting a new Pentecostal church not far from their trailer park. Although Bruce had not been raised in a particularly religious family, he agreed. Once inside the drab, echoing converted tractor shop, however, Jackie was embarrassed by the congregation. "They were singing, and swaying around, shouting 'Glory!' and 'Praise the Lord!'" But Bruce insisted they stay to the end of the service. Then the young minister called for sinners to repent. Like Rick, Bruce felt himself inexplicably propelled toward the altar. "I got about five steps, and I just hit an invisible *wall* or something," he remembers. He sank to his knees and began loudly praying, begging for repentance. Embarrassed, Jackie hung back, silent and confused.

Four days later, the minister led Bruce to the church's unlikely baptismal font, a converted industrial plate-dipping tank. He emerged from the water "speaking in tongues." Jackie was shocked to hear him chanting, his long hair streaming water, his eyes gleaming with a vigor she had never seen. That afternoon, Jackie approached the altar and knelt in repentance. She agreed to be baptized the next weekend. As the ceremony approached, she feared she was "too far gone for God to save." But when she stepped into the tepid water of the tank, she felt a strange force tingling throughout her body, lifting away the residual drug poison, washing her clean. "People used to ask if I was afraid of acid flashbacks," she says. "But after my baptism, I had no fear. I finally felt clean."

As often happens in such conversions, Bruce and Jackie threw themselves into the life of the church. Their Pentecostal denomination required worship several times a week. The congregation was a tight, perhaps claustrophobic, family. But the bonding provided the emotional support the young couple needed. The minister married them within a month.

His hair cut short, his eyes brightly focused, Bruce found a good job in an oil-rig company. The couple's first child, a boy they named Billy, was born a year after their conversion.

If Bruce and Jackie's story ended there, it would be just another testimonial of survival during the drug pandemic of the 1970s. But their conversion to Pentecostal Christianity was only the first step toward a new life.

His mind clear for the first time in years, Bruce felt a growing intellectual curiosity. The people at the church were kind, but few had more than a high school diploma. Bruce saw there was more to life for him than a factory job and church. He began night courses at a community college. Two years later, the couple was back in the Midwest, Bruce now a full-time engineering student. Jackie worked part-time and cared for their growing family, but she also found the energy to learn valuable skills in the technology of office automation. They still felt a spiritual void, however, so they joined a traditional Protestant church near the campus. Bruce earned an honors degree in a highly competitive branch of engineering and took a well-paid position in another Midwestern city.

One of the first things they did after the moving van left was to search for a new church. They have been members of this established Protestant congregation for almost fifteen years. Bruce is now a technical supervisor and Jackie manages an office. Their split-level home on a quiet cul-de-sac bears a predictable resemblance to the comfortable suburban houses they both knew as youngsters.

But as parents in the 1990s, Bruce and Jackie have no illusions about the dangers their three children face on these seemingly innocent Midwestern streets. Religion has become the solid foundation of their lives. They worship each week as a family; at each meal one of the kids says grace; family prayer is a nightly habit; and the children have all attended Sunday school and church summer camps. Bruce and Jackie spoke frankly about drugs to each of their children before they began middle school.

So far, the straightforward, unvarnished discussions seem to have worked. None of their children has given in to the temptation from the inevitable peer pressure to experiment that exists in every American community. And their parents' obvious concern is echoed in church-sponsored drug education.

Now a thoughtful, middle-age man with thinning hair, Bruce shakes his head when he considers how far he has come from that rented trailer littered with beer cans and plastic drug bongs. "I know religion can protect a family from drugs," he reflects, "but faith has to adapt with the times. You can't just shout and expect kids to listen. You have to provide a strong moral example, then be prepared to stay with them every inch of the way. Our faith helps us travel this road as a family."

Protecting Teenagers

Bruce's confidence in the protective ability of religiously grounded morality is supported by scientific research. As early as the 1970s, researchers found that the religious faith and practice of high school seniors in the Pacific Northwest—as reflected in their church attendance—significantly reduced their risk of becoming regular users of alcohol and marijuana. In that study, parental religious practice did not seem to be a protective factor. Young people's religious attendance did, however, seem to shield them from substance abuse.[19] And obviously, children raised in a religious home have a better chance of developing such protective faith than those growing up in a secular household.

An expanding body of research indicates that teenagers' religious faith is a highly significant factor in their turning away from drugs and alcohol, even if they have initially experimented.[20] Kenneth S. Kendler, a psychiatrist at the Medical College of Virginia, recently led a study of 1,902 adult twins that convincingly demonstrated that a devout religious life protects young adults from alcohol and nicotine addiction. Those with a strong faith drank and smoked less, and were at lower risk for problems associated with these behaviors.[21] And as Bruce and Jackie's hard-earned experience illustrates, a family does not have to devote an unreasonable amount of its week to organized religious worship for their adolescent children to be protected from alcohol and drug abuse.

Religion and Weight Control

I learned as a young family physician that illegal drugs and alcohol aren't the only "substances" that can damage our health. Too much rich food and not enough exercise can potentially be just as dangerous as Rick's little bags of heroin or Monty Cox's whiskey bottle. In fact, the office of the U.S. surgeon general recently warned Americans, "Obesity, a major public health problem in the United States, plays a central role" in the development of diabetes, and increases the risk of life-threatening high blood pressure, heart disease, certain cancers, and "all-cause mortality."[22] If you don't think many Americans are cutting short their lives with too much food and not enough exercise, take a close look at the people around you the next time you visit a shopping mall. But successful weight control has proven an elusive, frustrating goal for millions.

Anybody who's struggled with obesity knows that motivation and perseverance are vital aspects in any weight-control effort. And research finds that the support of a loving family or close-knit social community such as a religious congregation can bolster that motivation to persevere.[23]

Spiritually based weight-loss organizations are gaining popularity nationwide. Among the most effective are First Place and Prayer Walking.

First Place has helped tens of thousands of men and women in North America, Europe, and Asia. Participants are drawn from traditional and conservative Protestant, Roman Catholic, and Pentecostal congregations. Members meet weekly in time-tested small support groups, where motivational prayer and scriptural reading are emphasized. They also receive regular, practical low-fat recipes and exercise advice.

In First Place, the commitment essential to the often long effort needed for weight control rests solidly in individual faith. First Place draws on inspirational scriptural "memory verses," such as 1 Corinthians 12:27, "Now you are the body of Christ, and each of you is part of it." In emphasizing spiritual coping techniques, First Place and similar groups help calm the chronic anxiety that often underlies unhealthy eating habits. In fact, like Alcoholics Anonymous, the original spiritually based support group, First Place encourages tension-reducing prayer to ease the anguish that had been chronically soothed with food.[24]

Linus Mundy is the founder of the burgeoning Prayer Walking movement. In 1985, Mundy, who lives near a wooded state park in southern Indiana, found that vigorous hikes were more relaxing when combined with prayer. He also discovered that his combination of physical exercise and prayer gave him an unexpected sense of inner peace, which strengthened his resolve to lose weight. Mundy believes his program is ideal for today's busy people. "Action and contemplation have always been an American characteristic. By praying and walking at the same time, you really can get both spiritual and physical exercise."[25]

Parish Nursing

As I noted earlier, the parish nurse program is steadily growing in America. Only thirteen years ago, fewer than twenty nurses started a small organization to offer health screening and disease prevention to members of their congregations; today, more than three thousand nurses are active in the movement nationwide. Large congregations have the resources to hire a parish nurse full-time, but most churches rely on part-time or volunteer nurses. Parish nurses often supervise congregation health fairs that provide wellness information and free screening for high blood pressure, serum cholesterol, diabetes, and common cancers. Any physician will tell you that such regular screening is a major lifesaver, especially for older people. And, if someone seems to have dropped out of a congregation due to mounting depression, it is often the parish nurse who is the first health professional to sound the alarm.

The national Presbyterian Health Network has been involved in the parish nurse program since the 1980s. Hundreds of thousands of American Presbyterians can call on their parish nurses for health education, medical referrals, and vital, but often overlooked, patient advocacy support.

Deanna Koch is the parish nurse at the First Presbyterian Church in Muscatine, Iowa. "As a committed nurse and a Christian," she notes, "it's part of my stewardship to help with both the physical and spiritual needs of my church family."[26]

I'm a former nurse and understand the valuable contribution parish nurses are making in America's increasingly depersonalized health care system.

Health and Fanaticism

I'd be remiss if I ended this discussion of healthy lifestyles without directly addressing the problem of religious fanatics who use faith to justify depriving their families of health care, even when they are gravely ill. We have all seen media accounts of such tragic cases: Parents pray fervently for a dangerously sick child, but do not seek medical attention. Occasionally, emotionally unbalanced people with a twisted view of divine justice even starve a child for reasons they feel are divinely justified.[27]

As a physician, I have encountered patients who have cited religious reasons for stopping medication, not seeking timely medical care, or otherwise allowing their health to deteriorate for what mainstream religions would consider invalid or obscure reasons. Nationwide, the problem is often associated with extreme-fundamentalist congregations and with emotionally disturbed individuals. For example, members of the Faith Assembly in Indiana don't believe in prenatal care or physician-attended obstetrical delivery. Prior to intervention by the Indiana General Assembly in 1983 that largely stopped this practice, mothers and infants in this group suffered shockingly higher rates of maternal and infant mortality than those prevailing in Indiana (100 times and 3 times higher, respectively).[28] In Holland, a polio epidemic flared up because members of a religious group refused to vaccinate their children.[29]

I also have a colleague with a patient who suffers from advanced AIDS. She is newly married to a man who is HIV-negative. He insists on having unprotected intercourse with her, stating, "God will protect me."

Researchers from the University of California and advocates belonging to Children's Healthcare Is a Legal Duty (CHILD) studied the medical records of children who had died in the last twenty years following their parents' refusal of medical care. The researchers estimated probability of survival by comparing the cases to survival rates of children with similar problems whose parents did seek medical care. A total of 140 children, 81 percent of those who died, suffered conditions that normally had an excellent survival rate if care had been provided. In one shocking case, a two-year-old girl died an hour after choking on a banana while her parents frantically tried to assemble members of a religious circle to pray for the toddler.[30]

One of the most notorious examples of this practice was recently the subject of a 60 *Minutes* television report, which examined the family of Lorie and Dennis Nixon, members of a Faith Tabernacle congregation in Altoona, Pennsylvania. Fundamentalist Christians who believe in strictly literal biblical interpretation, the Nixons told CBS reporter Ed Bradley that they had never taken any of their numerous children to a doctor nor allowed any physical medication, even simple over-the-counter remedies.

Dennis Nixon stated that any form of modern medical intervention was against his family's rigid religious code. "The healing comes from God," he emphasized. "God's way is perfect."

Although most of their surviving eleven children have avoided life-threatening illness, their eight-year-old son Clayton died of complications of a common childhood ear infection in 1992, after his parents' prayer proved ineffective. Lorie and Dennis Nixon were convicted of involuntary manslaughter and received probation. In 1996, their sixteen-year-old daughter Shannon went into a diabetic coma, from which she did not respond to the ritual prayer that was offered in the place of modern medicine. When she died, Lorie and Dennis Nixon were again charged with involuntary manslaughter. After a conviction in a jury trial, a Pennsylvania judge sentenced them to serve up to five years in prison.

Reverend Charles Rush, the minister of nearby Christ Church, who has closely examined the religious implications of these tragic incidents, characterized the Nixons' actions as "spiritual malpractice." Rush noted that there is no biblical passage that forbids the faithful from seeking medical care.[31]

This is indeed a troubling story. But I must emphasize that the vast majority of fundamentalist Christians or ultraorthodox members of other faiths consider medical science one of God's benevolent creations, meant to prolong life and ease suffering. True, people with such beliefs often supplement medical intervention with intense private and congregational prayer or liturgical ceremony. However, they do not prevent their children from receiving inoculation against childhood diseases or other needed medical care.

Chapter Five

Religious People Cope Well with Stress

Those of you who surf the Internet might find it interesting to scan media archives for the key words "stress," "stressful," and "hectic" and that quaint old phrase, "rat race." And most of us over forty will agree that the demanding pace of life has accelerated inexorably since our own childhoods.

My psychiatric practice has made me aware that, for many people, the workplace has become a physically and emotionally exhausting marathon, exacerbated by the threat of downsizing layoffs. This chronic stress has robbed millions of the satisfaction and enjoyment they once felt at work. And simply reaching work each morning often means running a gauntlet of highways crammed with other stressed-out commuters, including an alarming number who vent their frustration through "road rage."

Other forms of stress are woven into the fabric of our affluent lifestyles. We suffer stress if we're deprived of the expensive furniture, appliances, or exotic vacations. And we succumb to stress when the mail carrier delivers a fresh stack of credit card bills, the inevitable aftermath of uncontrolled consumerism.

Stress can force us into tense isolation from our friends and family. Late-night television writers have mined a rich lode of dark comedy with sketches of families exploding with pent-up anger at the dinner table over trivial irritations. Are these skits funny? Sure. But the reason they are so popular is that they strike a chord of recognition in a nationwide audience.

The common stressors of our everyday lives can combine into an overwhelming negative synergy if we also suffer chronic physical illness.

Daily stress also might transform the normal pain of grief at the death of a loved one into crippling emotional agony.

Adolescence has never been easy. But today passing through the teenage years is all too often a wrenching emotional trauma. Violent street crime haunts millions of inner-city youth. Suicide has become one of the leading causes of death among adolescents and young adults, many from "safe" suburban homes.[1]

Research at Duke University and other institutions, however, reveals that religious people cope better with major stress events than those who lack the comfort of strong faith or the emotional support of a congregation. The basic elements that give meaning and purpose to the religious person's life are not easily threatened, even by dramatic life changes such as financial reverses, serious illness afflicting oneself or loved ones, or the death of a child or spouse. Because the annoyance and hectic pace of daily life do not threaten religious people's underlying values, their perceived stress levels are lower than those of the less religious. Faith helps mitigate the initial discouragement and hopelessness provoked by negative experience, which can steadily accumulate to debilitate people. As Khalita Jones exemplifies, faith nurtures the motivation and energy necessary to successfully cope with seemingly insurmountable hardship.

Alzheimer's disease, which emerged in the 1980s as a major health threat to people of middle age and older, also threatens the emotional well-being of victims' families. And, as our population ages, the devastation of Alzheimer's disease will mount proportionally.[2]

P. J. Burns's Story

Paul "P. J." Burns, seventy-nine, is a retired engineer who enjoyed a long, successful career with the Eastman Kodak Company in Kingsport, Tennessee. He and his wife, Lorene, eighty, raised three children and were active members of the First Baptist Church congregation. In the late 1980s, Lorene and P. J. looked forward to a busy, fulfilling "retirement." They planned to design and manage the construction of a tasteful upscale home development modeled on colonial Williamsburg.

"This was Lorene's project from the start," Paul Burns recalls. "She had the concept, she had the energy and concentration to work out the details, and she had the confidence to convince the bankers that the project was financially viable."

Only a few years into this demanding enterprise, however, Lorene's memory for details, once her strong asset, began to falter. "It started with repeating herself," Paul says. "But I just figured, *Well, we're both getting older, and we've got a lot on our minds.*" Then Lorene began to forget addresses and even friends' names. Still, Paul tried to deny her slow, but obvious, decline. His love for Lorene had grown to a deep bond since they'd married during World War II. *She'll snap back to her old self,* he thought.

Finally, their children insisted Paul seek medical help for Lorene. Dr. Marshal Folstein made the initial diagnosis that Lorene was suffering from Alzheimer's disease. The prominent New England psychiatrist is noted for his Folstein Mini-Mental State Exam, which had become standard worldwide among psychiatrists, neurologists, and general physicians as a tool for assessing persons with Alzheimer's. I first saw Lorene as a patient at the Duke University Geriatric Evaluation and Treatment (GET) Clinic. I was certain of Lorene's illness based on both the earlier diagnosis and my own observations. Now Paul had to confront the unquestioned reality of her condition. "It's very probable that your wife has Alzheimer's," I told Paul sadly one deceptively bright spring afternoon.

"But you're not one hundred percent sure?" Paul asked, melding hope with denial.

I shook my head and gently explained that only a postmortem examination could reveal a clinically certain diagnosis. But I had to add my realistic professional assessment: Lorene's condition would continue to deteriorate. She would probably enjoy stable periods, but she would not recover any of the mental acuity she had already lost. Soon, Lorene would have to enter a nursing home. Alzheimer's was a terminal illness; she would never recover.

All his adult life, Paul had dealt with the complex challenges of engineering, a profession that routinely solved even the most complicated problems. He was used to working hard and obtaining results. But sitting in that sunlit doctor's office, Paul was confronted with the harsh fact that Lorene's illness was beyond his control.

Paul took his wife back to Tennessee and launched headlong into the backlogged work on the new home development. But without Lorene, the project had lost its appeal. Paul and his wife had shared their lives for almost fifty years. Now Lorene was drifting away, and he could do nothing to rescue her.

Soon, Lorene needed full-time care. A careful planner, Paul had decided to close their home in Kingsport and move Lorene into a North Carolina nursing home where she could be treated by Alzheimer's specialists. But before that final move, he wanted to take her for one last summer weekend with the family at their beach house on Kiawah Island, on the South Carolina coast.

As they drove over the familiar humpbacked bridges above the sunny coastal marsh, Lorene smiled in vague recognition. But Paul gripped the steering wheel, raw and agitated. The emotional strain of such situations can assume many forms. Paul's reaction to this stress was churning, angry frustration. He found the smiling crowd of grandchildren at the house suddenly intolerable. And the beach house itself, a sanctuary that Lorene had loved so much, seemed cold, alien. Later, Paul strode off alone to the weathered plank stairs on the dunes overlooking the flat expanse of tidal beach. But he found no peace in the creaming surf or the gulls' graceful flight.

All his life he had worked for Lorene and the family. He had been a good husband, a devoted father. For five decades, he had dreamed of a prosperous, active retirement with Lorene. Now she was condemned to the prison of her illness. Some days, her eyes would warm with recognition that he was her husband. But when he came home on many afternoons, she would smile politely, seeing him as just another kindly stranger visiting the house.

"Why?" he growled between clenched teeth, his tone a harsh surprise. He was rudely demanding an answer, speaking directly to God without the intervening formality of prayer. Paul knew he did not deserve such a punishment. "Why us? Why *me?*" The surf rolled in; the gulls wheeled in the bright sunlight. He heard no answer.

Then his son Steven came down the sandy stairs. "Can I pray for you, Dad?" Steven asked, placing his hand on Paul's shoulder. Paul reached back, his vision clouded with tears, and gripped Steven's hand. As they prayed, Paul gradually warmed with a reassuring peace that washed away the chill anger, like the Gulf Stream surf smoothing the beach.

This, he saw, was the life that God had given them. Paul and Lorene, their family, this beach and ocean, the entire complex world, all this existed by the grace of God. Lorene's illness was part of God's larger plan, which Paul knew he could never grasp in this lifetime. There could be no other response to the question, "Why?" Paul knew he must not continue to flail around in self-pity, desperately searching for ways to change his life. Instead, he saw, God now wanted him to do his best for Lorene and to help others whose lives were so much harder than his own.

It was time to move Lorene to the nursing home and make the best of life. Once Paul himself was settled in a nearby retirement apartment complex that boasted a fitness center and well-equipped hobbyist workshop, however, he still suffered bouts of chill loneliness. Daily tasks such as shopping and housekeeping were often unreasonably irritating.

But when Paul joined the large and dynamic First Baptist Church congregation near his new home in North Carolina for help, his stressful isolation slowly disappeared. Church members regularly visited Lorene, bringing flowers for her room, bright cards on holidays replete with the scrawled signatures of Sunday school children, and small treats of candy. When the weather was good, they strolled with her on the grounds of the nursing home. Paul saw he was not alone in his struggle with Lorene's illness.

"It's such a blessing, knowing these new friends really care about her," Paul told Steven.

Over the coming years, as Lorene's condition declined, Paul's spiritual strength grew. He had been a dutiful member of his church in Kingsport for over forty years, but he had never felt deeply for people suffering the pain of illness or bereavement until he himself had tasted this pain. Now Paul sought them out. For the first time in his successful life, he understood that true achievement came from relieving pain in others. At church, among other retired people, and even during chance encounters with strangers, Paul found he could now recognize unspoken anguish. "Somehow, I can see people in silent pain," Paul explains, "those who have deep needs but can't express them."

Paul now prays every day, but never simply to relieve his own pain, as he once did. When he heard that a friend had been diagnosed with a terminal illness, Paul took the time to seek him out. "I just want you to know I'm praying for you," Paul explained, arriving unannounced after a long drive.

The friend was deeply touched. Men of their generation had learned to muffle such open compassion.

Paul's concern for the afflicted has brought him unexpected personal comfort. He has befriended patients at Lorene's nursing home whose illness has been far crueler than hers. One woman's dementia is so severe that she often becomes agitated in the dining room, shouting unintelligibly at other patients and the staff. The first time Paul witnessed the outburst, he rose from the table and softly sang "Amazing Grace," his face close to her ear. The familiar words and rhythm of the hymn immediately calmed her. Now whenever the woman becomes agitated during one of Paul's visits, all he has to do is sing the opening verses of the hymn and she closes her eyes, smiles peacefully, and rocks in silent accompaniment.

Paul has joined a volunteer group of retired men who work all year making wooden toys as Christmas gifts for disadvantaged children. He specializes in sturdy, brightly painted toy trucks. The days he spends in his workshop, hunched over the band saw and power sander, handling the smooth chunks of Carolina pine, are as satisfying to Paul as anything he accomplished during his long professional career. Each December, Paul and his fellow volunteers personally deliver the toys to shelters and day-care centers.

Last year, Paul was just sitting down to unpack his bag of toys when a toddler clomped across the floor, crawled into his lap, and pressed her face against his chest. Lorene had always loved being among small children at Christmas. Now, hugging this lonely toddler, who had no sense of their differences in race or class but only sought a moment of comforting warmth, Paul recognized a divine intention in this brief human exchange. God, he believed, had brought Lorene and him together so many years before so that he would be here now to guide her through her long illness. In turn, the pain of Lorene's suffering had tapped a hidden wellspring of compassion within Paul that he was now able to draw upon to comfort others, like this child.

Once, the stress of Lorene's condition had driven Paul to anguished despair. Today he feels a sense of fulfillment he would have never known had he not made this painful spiritual journey.

Stress and Religious Faith: Maton's Study

I could use the jargon of the mental health profession to describe Paul Burns's odyssey as "successful coping" with an unacceptably painful level of stress. But such bland scientific terms disguise a far richer, more complex experience. And there is mounting research evidence to suggest that drawing on religious faith as a shield against intense stress might be the *most* effective tactic in our emotional repertoire. In 1985, for example, a study of coping among 240 people caring for loved ones with Alzheimer's disease found that those who saw their burden within a spiritual context faced their situations with a more positive attitude than caregivers who were less spiritually oriented.[3]

In the late 1980s, University of Maryland psychologist Kenneth I. Maton examined the role of strong personal faith ("spiritual support") as a buffer against serious stress.[4] Maton compared the religious coping (dependence on religious faith to relieve psychological stress) of recently bereaved parents in a support group and freshmen at an East Coast university undergoing painful stress in their adjustment to higher education and life away from home. In both groups, the people with the strongest religious faith appeared to be best shielded from depression caused by stress. For example, parents who had lost a child and who answered yes to the statement "I experience God's love and caring on a regular basis" were better protected against the agonizing stress of bereavement than their counterparts who did not have such emotionally fulfilling faith.

The college freshmen under stress who affirmed "My religious faith helps me to cope during times of difficulty" also handled stress better than those for whom religion was less important. Attendance at religious service, which usually provides social support, was not a significant factor among the college students suffering from stress.[5]

This research indicates that the more painful the stress, the more comfort people discover in their faith. I also find the study interesting because of the diversity of the subjects—parents who have lost children and young people having difficulty coping with the adult world.

I've already noted that the breakup of a marriage through divorce can be almost as stressful as the death of a child. Although there aren't yet firm research findings, I feel certain that the emotional strain people such as Paul Burns suffer helplessly watching their lifelong spouse slide into the irreversible dementia of Alzheimer's disease can be almost as severe.

The lesson of Maton's research seems to be that faith can heal intense emotional distress, regardless of its source. And, the greater the emotional pain experienced by people such as Paul Burns, the more benefit they receive from their religious faith.

Mainstream Stress-Busters: The Duke University Study

Given my long interest in the health of elderly people, I led a study on religion as a coping strategy among older adults early in my research career at Duke. Our subjects were men and women with a mean educational level of 12.6 years, which was high for their peer group and indicated that many had university degrees. They completed questionnaires on their methods of coping with the most stressful events in their recent experience, in the previous ten years, and over their entire lives. Reliance on religious faith was the most frequently mentioned coping technique, particularly among women. Three-quarters of the people who relied on religion to cope with stress mentioned that they placed trust in God, prayed, or obtained emotional strength from God.[6]

We purposely selected relatively better-educated and financially secure older adults (similar to Paul Burns) in order to assess the importance of religious coping among people who had obviously led successful lives by secular standards. Our finding that faith provided such strong emotional comfort to these people contrasts sharply with the once-widespread assumption in the medical profession (often echoed in popular-entertainment images) that it is typically marginal, insecure people, driven by failure, who seek comfort in religion.[7]

Chronic Illness and Religious Faith: Genie's Story

During my clinical psychiatric practice, I've met a number of people who have successfully drawn on their religious faith to relieve the stress caused by chronic, severe physical illness. Genie Lewis, an emotionally and spiritually mature woman in her forties, recently related one of the most amazing accounts of the healing power of faith that I have ever heard. She has kindly permitted me to tell her inspiring story in this book.

In the early 1980s, when Genie was in her thirties, she began to suffer unexplainable pain in her back and limbs, followed by bouts of debilitating fatigue. Some of the doctors Genie consulted diagnosed arthritis. Others frankly admitted they were stumped. Genie, who had married and divorced in her twenties and was now engaged again, tried to ignore her increasingly frequent symptoms.

Then, in 1988, she woke up one morning feeling drained and groggy. When she dragged her legs out of bed, she was shocked to find that her feet and legs were completely numb from toes to hip and that she had no feeling of contact with the floor. Grabbing with her right hand to throw back the covers, she saw three fingers twisted into a numb claw. Genie was seized by fear. "Am I going to die?" she moaned.

That episode sparked another round of unsuccessful diagnoses. The numbness was episodic, passing through a spectrum that ranged from actual paralysis to mobility that was accompanied by fiery, shooting agony. Genie spent days hunched painfully in specialists' waiting rooms or stretched out on examination tables. She underwent multiple scans and painful neuroelectrical stimulation tests that seemed more like torture than a modern medical procedure. Although Genie had always considered herself a religious person and Stanley, her fiancé, was a Christian family counselor, she began to feel that God had abandoned her.

Well-intentioned friends offered spiritual advice. "You'll find real comfort in the Bible," one woman suggested, handing Genie an annotated book of scriptural advice. Genie accepted the Bible with faint thanks. But inside, she was seething. *I don't want a book. I want a cure.*

Eventually, the neurologists reached a grim consensus: Genie Lewis was suffering a severe, atypical form of multiple sclerosis. She understood that her condition was chronic and that the medical profession could only treat her symptoms, not the underlying disorder. Genie had always been energetic and upbeat. Now her world had shrunk to a dark tunnel of hopeless pain. Her right side was the most seriously affected area. Sometimes the burning jolts of pain in her right elbow and rib cage were so intense it felt as if some unseen device was ripping the arm from the socket. During these episodes, even narcotic painkillers had little effect. Genie was virtually held prisoner in the agonizing confines of her body, unable to work or perform simple tasks during the most severe occurrences.

Then, inexplicably, the pain would disappear. It was during such a remission that she and Stanley married and enjoyed several uninterrupted months of happiness. But Genie knew the agony was only hidden, lurking to spring another attack. The stress of waiting was almost as severe as the pain. She became withdrawn from Stanley and other members of her family. As much as she hated the stupor of the Demerol and morphine, at least the drugs temporarily numbed her jangled emotion.

Years passed, with her symptoms steadily growing worse. Now the pain spread down her spine. Racked by severe spasms, she developed an unnatural curvature to her spinal column, which provoked degenerative arthritis in her vertebrae and hips. Genie underwent painful spinal surgery and became dependent on massive steroid injections and increasingly heavy doses of narcotics to hold the pain at bay.

By the summer of 1997, Genie felt she had been driven past the brink of insanity. There was almost no part of her body untouched by pain. Trying to walk, her feet burned, as if she was walking on hot coals. Her back was so sensitive that she couldn't lie in bed. But her doctors concluded there was nothing to be gained from further hospital care.

There were days when Genie felt trapped and gripped by guilt because she was immobilized by pain and Stanley had to perform all the cooking, cleaning, and laundry after he had worked all day.

I've got nowhere to run, she thought bleakly one hot summer night when the rest of the family was sleeping.

Genie moved to an armchair, where she could sometimes find a comfortable position.

She spotted the Bible on an end table. It looked like a dead black stone, devoid of any human comfort. *God,* she moaned silently, *You're the only one who can help me.* But Genie felt no relief. "If the rest of my life will be like this," she muttered, "it really is not worth living."

Overwrought, Genie was feeling increasingly isolated from Stanley and the other members of her family. Early one afternoon, perched exhausted in her armchair, she dragged the Bible into her lap and scanned the pages lethargically. Her eye fell to a chapter head: Hebrews 11, Verse 1. "Now faith is the assurance of things hoped for, the conviction of things not seen."

Genie snapped back into conscious focus and read the passage again. She had often seen the verse, but had never felt that it applied to her. Now a presence more intense than her pain, more soothing than the narcotics, grew inside her. She believed it was the Holy Spirit speaking directly to her inner self. "I have placed a healing substance within you," the silent voice intoned. "Soon I will release it."

Genie felt a spark of optimistic peace. Then the pain crackled through her body. "Healing substance . . . ," she whispered scornfully. "Sure. What else are you selling today?"

By evening, the pain and spasms became so severe that her right fingers clamped on to the book in her lap and she had to pry them loose. Bending to the effort, her back was seized with agony. *It will be a real miracle if I see tomorrow,* she realized with resigned insight, *because I sure can't take much more of this.*

Late that night, Genie finally slipped into a deep sleep she had not enjoyed for weeks. When the dream began, the images were so crisply vivid that Genie was convinced she had entered another level of reality.

She was a girl of fourteen again, her body young and supple, free of pain. This teenager was overwhelmed with joyful optimism, strolling along a neat pathway between wide, sunlit lawns and gardens in a beautifully landscaped park. But she saw no other people. Looking up from the flowers, Genie confronted a high wrought-iron gate, the only portal in a tall, featureless wall that curved away to the horizon. A brilliant radiance swelled behind the gate, brighter than any light she'd ever seen, yet not painful. "Where is this light coming from?" Genie's young voice asked. She was curious, not afraid. Then she noticed that the gate stood ajar.

Squinting, Genie saw that the path climbed beautifully through wooded hills dotted with graceful stone buildings beyond the wall. She smiled with curiosity at the charming landscape. Then she heard a deep, rustling sound like wind in the trees. Her mind was flooded with a profound calm that brought with it a wisdom Genie had never imagined possible. She recognized the nature of the dream, sensing the consciousness of her teenage persona within her afflicted adult body. A voice spoke with gentle, loving clarity. "If you want to, you may step over."

Still completely calm, Genie's mind opened to encompass both her twisted form in the chair and her healthy younger self poised at the gate, all surrounded by the peaceful brilliance. *This is really Jesus,* she thought. Genie understood she was in the presence of the Jesus she had prayed to as a young girl, innocent of any knowledge of how pain and bitterness would one day warp her life. God was offering her relief, infinite peace. All she had to do was slide open that gate and step across the threshold.

Then she was aware of the voice once more. "You can still go back." It was not a command, but a kindly suggestion, a choice. Genie knew she could end her suffering with a simple step. Or she could return and accept the life she had been given. The girl with straight, muscular limbs turned gracefully and strode back down the path, her back turned to the radiance.

Genie woke completely in the armchair. "He's given me a chance at life." The words came automatically, spoken with unquestionable certainty. Genie realized that God cared enough for her that he had prepared a place of infinite, peaceful healing, should she choose to go there. But there was still work to do here on earth.

Shifting her limbs cautiously, Genie felt more gratification than surprise that the usual spasms of agony did not assault her. *I will be better now*, she thought. Certainly not perfect, not fully liberated from pain, but well enough to complete the work she had been given.

The next morning, Genie found herself walking almost steadily around the house. For the first time in months, she did not need to swallow painkillers to face the simple tasks of bathing and dressing. It was almost as if the healthy teenage girl of the dream had taken residence within her withered middle-age body.

Over the coming months, Genie remained virtually free of pain. Her energy returned. Her ragged emotions grew whole and focused. Genie's doctors were amazed at her recovery.

I listened closely to her story, searching for words and phrases indicative of a drug-induced hallucination or delirium provoked by chronic pain. But I found none. I have no doubt that Genie's dream was as vivid and healing as she described. Was it a valid case of divine intervention? Neither I nor any other scientific researcher has the skills to answer that question.

But medical science can chart her remarkable improvement. Months into her inexplicable recovery, Genie Lewis has dramatically longer periods free of pain than she ever enjoyed in the past. She has reduced her medications to a fraction of her previous regimen, and weaned herself off all narcotic analgesics. Yet she has not experienced a "miraculous" cure of her underlying physical illness. Genie still suffers from multiple sclerosis with severe complications. In fact, she recently developed stress fractures in her feet and was confined to uncomfortable foot casts for weeks.

But after the profound spiritual experience of the dream, Genie Lewis is able to cope with her illness with remarkably calm acceptance. "Every person on earth has some heavy burden to carry," she said recently. "God showed me the way to cope with mine."

Today, Genie works as a cocounselor in Stanley's practice. She is more certain than ever that her adolescent dream persona made the correct decision in turning away from the radiant peace to complete the work of her adult life.

Has Genie's faith *healed* her illness? Not in the strict medical sense of the term. But does her multiple sclerosis and its cruel sequelae continue to dominate Genie Lewis's life? The answer is certainly no. Genie has achieved a level of emotional tranquillity through her faith that I believe many mental health professionals would profit from studying.

And research continues to substantiate the importance of religious faith as a personal resource in coping with the painful stress of physical illness. In 1992 and 1998, we published studies in the *American Journal of Psychiatry* and the *International Journal of Geriatric Psychiatry* presenting findings that a significant number of patients rely on religious faith to mitigate the stress engendered by their physical afflictions.[8,9]

The Religious Coping Index (RCI)

Working with colleagues, I helped develop a Religious Coping Index (RCI) that we administered to hospitalized patients with serious medical illness. The RCI is made up of three items: an open-ended coping question ("What enables you to cope?"), a self-rating by the patient, and a separate rating by a trained interviewer (based on a brief discussion of how the patient uses religion to cope).

When we used this index in studies of hospitalized patients, we found that between 24 and 42 percent of older people spontaneously mentioned religion when asked what enabled them to cope with their illness.

Asked to rate on a scale of 0 to 10 to what extent they used religion to cope with emotional distress, approximately 90 percent of the patients indicated they relied on their religious faith at least to a moderate degree, and almost 70 percent said they used religious coping to a large extent or more.

During the interviews, examiners asked patients for examples of their religious coping, then rated them on a scale of 0 to 10, based on a judgment of how much they depended on religion to help cope with the stress of illness. Between one-half and two-thirds received ratings of 7.5 or higher, indicating a large extent of religious coping. The resulting three-item index produced total scores ranging from 0 to 30.

Hospitalized patients who rated highest on the RCI showed the lowest levels of depression, indicating they were coping well with the stress of their illness.[10] This was particularly true among the severely disabled. Religious coping scores also proved to be a good predictor of lower depression levels six months after hospital discharge, a further indication that religious faith helps protect people from stress.[11]

What I find most significant in this evidence is that severely ill patients who trust in God and pray acquire an indirect sense of control over their illness. This is probably because they are certain God is personally interested in them and answers their prayers.

Certainly, Genie Lewis acquired such trust during her intense personal religious experience that centered on her remarkable dream.

This research reveals something about the impact of severe physical illness on religious people. When they become sick or disabled, many people angrily blame God for their suffering. Others turn to Him for comfort. Initial anger and questioning directed at God—Paul Burns's anguished, "Why *me?*"—usually resolves, however, and people find comfort in their faith.

Compliance and Control

The degree to which patients draw comfort from religion has a lot to do with their sense of control in their lives, which in turn influences their vital, but often intangible, level of cooperation in treatment, i.e., joining in physical therapy, following medication regimens, etc. It is well established that depressed patients are less compliant. Since religious faith helps people cope with stress and avoid depression, it is probably useful for clinicians to assess their patients' level of religious coping.

Certainly a perceived sense of mastery over illness bolsters people's quality of life, even among the severely disabled. I'm often reminded of a woman in her eighties who suffered a major stroke that left her almost completely paralyzed (a neurologic condition known as the "locked-in" syndrome). Although she was alert, she had motor control only over her eyelids. During a visit, her pastor complained that he had so many prayer requests for ill members of the congregation that he simply did not have time to answer them. "Will you help me out and pray for some of them?" he asked. The paralyzed woman blinked twice to agree. She began her prayer routine immediately. This brought her a great sense of inner peace and satisfaction, especially when members of her church visited and commented on how her prayers had been answered. Although she only lived a few more months, she remained cheerful and fulfilled to the end.

I find her story a heartening example of the healing power of faith. A person in her condition had every logical reason for anxious despair. But she learned that no matter how intractable her physical disability, she still possessed the strength to serve God. If you have seen as many depressed older people hospitalized for physical illness as I have, I'm sure you'd agree that delivering such inner peace to many of these suffering individuals is still beyond the ability of medical science.

Courage and Optimism: Peggy's Story

A seriously ill person doesn't have to be hospitalized with a crippling disability to enjoy the coping benefits of religious faith. To see Peggy La Vigne, an energetic woman with silver-gray hair, her face adorned in gaudy clown's makeup and Chaplinesque attire, on her way to cheer up shut-ins and nursing home residents in New Bern, North Carolina, you'd never know she has endured several life-threatening conditions. Indeed, Peggy has had a harrowing life by secular standards.

In the 1960s, when she divorced her husband, Peggy had two small sons to raise alone. One night, her two-year-old boy woke her asking for a glass of milk. When she opened a hallway door, she found the house shrouded in choking white smoke. Half the small frame bungalow was already engulfed in flames. And the corridor to the baby's room was flooding with suffocating smoke. Then she sensed a bright sphere hovering near her face that somehow led her to his room.

Choking and half-blinded, she managed to rip open a screen and drop the toddler and the baby into the cushioning branches of a large bush.

Amid the terror and confusion of the fire, Peggy hadn't had time to think about the strange light that had guided her through the smoke. But, as the fire trucks sprayed water into the gutted frame house, she trembled with the realization of the events she and her children had just survived. Her two-year-old had never before woken her late to ask for milk. And how could she ever account for that glowing sphere that had led her to the baby's crib? "He was there with me," Peggy said in awe, realizing that God had sent his angels to protect her and the two little boys. *God is involved in my life*, she recognized. Peggy understood that she could put her complete faith and trust in God, regardless of the challenge she faced.

Her trust in divine providence has never been shaken since then, despite ongoing troubles. Peggy entered the job market at a time when divorced mothers received little encouragement. But she worked steadily, advancing from clerical jobs to managerial responsibilities. Early in her career, however, she learned she had dangerous atherosclerosis, made worse by apparently intractable high blood pressure.

Peggy turned to prayer, starting a weekly luncheon prayer group at her office. As a young child, she had been taught that Jesus Christ could become a personal friend in time of need, that prayer and Bible study enabled people to surmount obstacles. Now Peggy gave herself over completely to Jesus Christ, accepting Him as her personal friend and savior. She took this personal conversion seriously, making amends with everyone she might have offended and offering forgiveness to all those who might have offended her. She decided the best way to practice her religion was to live the lessons of the Bible.

In 1987, Peggy underwent surgery for breast cancer. As the anesthesia took hold, she felt a warmth spreading through the sterile operating room. "This cancer will never bother you again," an inner voice assured her.

Then, in 1992, Peggy was sent to Duke University Medical Center, where her oldest son was now an intern. A complicated diagnostic procedure finally revealed a life-threatening vascular blockage in her stomach. Peggy faced highly invasive vascular graft surgery, which required "roundtable" consultations among the members of her care team. I know from clinical experience that many people with her combination of physical problems would suffer extreme psychological stress facing such an operation. But Peggy was almost serene the morning of her surgery. As her son helped wheel her into the operating room, she spoke to her Lord in almost conversational prayer. "It really doesn't matter whether I stay here or go up to be with You," she said. "I accept whichever way You prefer, Lord. But You know my son is getting married in eight months and he'd be very disappointed if his mother was not sitting in that first pew."

Peggy survived the surgery and endured a long and painful recovery. She is convinced her faith was the largest single factor in this healing.

This experience prepared her for another grave medical crisis a few years later. She twice suffered severe internal hemorrhaging of unknown origin, but recovered with her optimistic outlook undampened. Recently Peggy La Vigne was diagnosed with atrial fibrillation, which often produces bouts of extreme fatigue. She finds she can reenergize herself by calling her close prayer friend, Betty. Praying and reading scripture together over the telephone relaxes Peggy and she finds she can drift off into healing sleep.

Peggy has unshakable faith that God remains in complete control of her life and is capable of "fixing" any of her medical problems.

Today Peggy belongs to two congregations, a traditional Episcopal church where she receives communion every Sunday and a charismatic church where she attends emotionally intimate worship service.

Several times a week, she worships privately with prayer "warriors," studying biblical passages for relevance in her life, as well as praying for others.

I believe Peggy La Vigne is an excellent example of certain people who have achieved mastery of their emotions during extended periods of stress brought on by physical illness. Peggy is convinced that God has intervened repeatedly in her life, and this bolsters her with a sense of control over her physical condition. Referring to scripture, Peggy describes her hopeful serenity in the face of ongoing health problems: "I fear not, for God has given me a spirit of power."

Religious Coping: Pargament's Study

Peggy La Vigne is virtually a textbook example of successful religious coping. My friend Kenneth I. Pargament, Ph.D., a psychology professor at Bowling Green State University in Ohio and author of *The Psychology of Religion and Coping,* is the world's pioneering researcher in this field.[12]

He and his colleagues conducted a landmark study of religious coping techniques used by members of Midwestern churches who had faced serious negative events in their own lives or in those of close friends or family members. These problems included illness or injury, either their own or their loved ones'; death of a close friend or loved one; marital strife such as separation or divorce; or professional problems such as being laid off or fired. The researchers wanted to establish with a degree of scientific certainty whether anecdotal accounts that religious people cope better with stress than their less religious counterparts were valid.[13]

After a rigorous analysis of data from a sample of 586 people who belonged to mainline Protestant and Catholic churches, as well as to less traditional nondenominational congregations, Pargament's team published its findings. A highly significant 78 percent of the people studied used their religious faith in coping with problems. Some drew on a larger spiritual context, perhaps God's overall plan for their lives, to give meaning to negative situations and provide emotional strength. Many were shielded from stress by "a recognition of the limits of [their] personal agency (e.g., 'Took control over what I could and gave the rest up to God')."[14] People with this outlook were clearly protected from the emotional damage of intense stress. The researchers also found that involvement with "religious rituals," attendance at religious services, prayer, focusing on scripture, and consciously trying to lead a more moral, loving life also helped people cope with stress, as did seeking spiritual comfort from the clergy and members of the congregation.

I think one of the most significant findings of the study was the comparison of religious and nonreligious "avoidance" coping techniques. In this context, avoidance means mentally focusing on something other than the stressful problem. Remember, classical psychology rooted in Freudian thought has long held that religion is a type of escapist delusion that prevents an emotionally mature person from confronting reality. However, Pargament's study established that people who seek comfort in religion during stressful times have better emotional outcomes than those who rely on nonreligious avoidance techniques.

I believe it's time for clinicians treating chronic physical disorders, such as those Peggy La Vigne suffers, and for mental health professionals to reconsider the important role of religious faith in coping with the stressful experiences we all encounter in life.

African-Americans and Religious Coping: The Michigan Study

African-Americans have historically had to deal with the stress of racial discrimination, rural and urban poverty, and, in recent years, the violent crime plaguing our inner cities. But many of them have shown an amazing ability to cope with such stress. During my family practice and geriatric training in the Midwest and North Carolina, I often observed a marked tranquillity among older black patients. I also noticed that these elderly men and women often made references to the role of God and faith in their lives. Did religion shield them from the emotionally damaging stress of discrimination, poverty, and crime-plagued neighborhoods?

University of Michigan researchers Neal Krause and Thanh Van Tran studied a nationwide sample of elderly black Americans to determine whether their religious faith helped buffer them against the emotionally harmful effects of stressful events in their lives.[15] While noting that the black church has historically provided an emotional haven, Krause and Van Tran offered rigorously analyzed data to show the degree to which membership in a black congregation protected people from harmful stress: ". . . while stress tends to erode feelings of mastery and self-esteem, these negative effects are offset or counterbalanced by religious involvement [in black churches]," the authors concluded. They might have been describing the invaluable contribution Deliverance Evangelistic Church and congregations like it have made in the lives of millions of African-Americans.

Suicide and the Faith Factor: Chris's Story

I probably don't have to remind parents of teenagers that suicide and other self-destructive acts of violence are serious threats to their families. Suicide now ranks as the third-leading cause of death among young people fifteen to twenty-four years old, behind accidents and homicide.[16]

The basic principles of human psychology teach us that suicide is almost always an act of despair stemming from depression, which in turn is often engendered by unbearable stress. And the grim progression from stress to depression to suicide among adolescents and young adults has accelerated in the last three decades. In 1960, for example, the per-100,000 suicide rate for adolescents fifteen to nineteen years old was 5.6. In 1980, this rate had zoomed to 13.3 per 100,000.[17] Tragically, the suicide rate for adolescents and young adults has fallen only slightly since its peak in the late 1970s. Additionally, researchers have pointed out that a certain percentage of car accident deaths may be suicides, so self-destructive behavior by young people might be even more prevalent than statistics indicate.

Today, few mental health professionals doubt that depression is a growing threat to America's young people. University of Pennsylvania psychologist Martin E. P. Seligman, the recently elected president of the American Psychological Association, has led research into the alarming growth of depression among young Americans. Seligman has documented that depression in children has relentlessly increased during this century. About 1 percent of children born around World War I (1917–18 for the U.S.) suffered depression; by World War II, the childhood depression rate had tripled to 3.5 percent. Seligman estimates that about 12 to 15 percent of high school graduates today suffer significant levels of depression.[18]

I believe the story of a young man named Chris Benfield provides an excellent and moving example of how religious faith can protect troubled adolescents who are struggling with stress-induced depression and are at increased risk of committing suicide. Chris has generously agreed to share his experience in this book, but I have changed the names of his friends to protect their privacy. Although Chris was raised in the anonymous suburban sprawl of the New South during the prosperity of the past two decades, his story will seem painfully familiar to families across the country.

Chris was born in 1978, the second son in a large family. His parents struggled to provide a decent home, but were buffeted by the uncertainties of the boom-and-recession roller coaster that has dominated the region. But although they couldn't provide the luxuries common to more affluent families, Chris's parents were loving, concerned, and religious. They belonged to a supportive charismatic church that stressed morality and godliness over secular achievement.

Early in childhood, however, Chris began to question the place of religion in his life. Although he seemed a bright, active child, Chris performed poorly in the classroom. Teachers labeled him "slow." After repeated failures in the early grades, he was diagnosed with dyslexia and attention deficit disorder. Chris was shunted into a special-education track, which drew the cruel taunts of his classmates.

By sixth grade, Chris was so angry and embarrassed at the other kids'
teasing that he was "weird" that he would enter the school playground
each morning with his jaw clenched and his stomach burning and
knotted tight. That year he lashed out in anger, beating anyone who
dared mock him. His parents took Chris out of the crowded public system and experimented unsuccessfully with home schooling. He often
tried to escape stress by hiking into the nearby woods to practice "survival" skills.

When Chris tried public education again in high school, he was
even more emotionally isolated, desperate for acceptance, hungry for
friendship. As in many parts of the South, high school cliques formed
around team sports and prestigious churches. Rejected by the socially
successful kids, Chris sought out other troubled youngsters from among
the "alternative" subculture that embraced anarchy like a religion.
Now he wore only black, drank beer in daily binges, smoked marijuana,
and plunged into a depressive spiral centered on "death metal" rock.
Drunk one aimless afternoon in a mall, he had his left eyebrow pierced
and adorned with a studded ring, his "screw the world" statement. He
and his friends spent hours hunched around high-decibel boom boxes,
ranting the "dry lung" lyrics of their favorite groups. The music focused
on violence, alienation, and the ultimate liberation: suicide.

Expelled from school, Chris withdrew to his room, almost hypno-
tized by the repetitive cacophony of the "industrial death" blasting
from his stereo. No school, no church, no decent people would ever
take him back, Chris knew. He threw his knives until the bedroom wall
was chewed open to the house frame. Then he completed the destruction with his bleeding fists.

"You'll be eighteen soon," Chris's father told him one night, his
voice utterly defeated. "Then I'm afraid you'll just have to leave home.
We can't keep you here to influence the younger kids."

A few weeks later, Chris was drinking with "Jim," a kid who drifted
on the fringes of the alternative group. Jim suddenly dropped his beer
can and announced that the world made "no fucking sense." He staggered home, found a gun, and shot himself. The boy's grave became an
unofficial pilgrimage site where other disturbed youngsters would

drink, smoke dope, then "mosh" like zombies to their bleak music.

Chris was shocked by Jim's suicide, but understood his desperation. No matter how hard Chris tried to win acceptance, he always seemed to hit a wall of scorn and rejection. *I'm gonna die soon myself,* he realized. *And I'll never get to heaven, living like I do.* This insight only deepened his depression.

Somehow, his parents persuaded Chris to give high school another try. He was repeating his junior year when "Bill," a boy from the alternative scene, came to the house seeking a place to sleep. Bill's parents were dragging out a bitter divorce; there was only noisy hatred at home. "Maybe Jim had the right idea," Bill said. "Just leave all this shit behind."

Chris thought about his own struggle with incomprehensible world history and geometry textbooks, about the giggles and sneers he endured each day from the good Christian jocks and cheerleaders in the school corridors. Bill was probably right: Why face the shit each day? Chris was about to mouth an instinctively cynical comment when he heard the back porch screen door squeak close—his dad coming home late after working. Despite his troubles, Chris slowly realized, his parents had always worked hard to preserve a loving home. And much of that warmth was grounded in their simple, unshakable faith in God. How could he betray them through suicide? Chris teetered with confusion, on the verge of asking Bill to pray with him, to ask God to ease their anguish. But that would be too "uncool," Chris knew. Instead, he simply offered Bill the refuge of his parents' house.

Two mornings later, Chris's high school principal approached him outside of study hall. "A boy named Bill dropped this off for you," he said, handing over an envelope. An old grade school basketball medal and an enamel tourist pin from the Smoky Mountains were folded into a sheet of paper torn from a notebook.

"This stuff means a lot to me," Bill's note said. "It's for you, Chris. You're my best, my *only* friend. I can't take any more. Don't be angry for what I'm going to do . . ."

"My God," Chris shouted, "he's really going to kill himself."

He asked the principal to drive them to the cemetery where Jim was buried. They found the distinctive tire tracks of Bill's pickup truck in the muddy red clay. "We're too late," Chris moaned.

He dashed into a nearby thicket, seeking refuge as he had when he was a lonely, taunted child. Then he had prayed to a loving Jesus, begging that the other children stop teasing him and be his friend. When Bill had mentioned suicide two nights before, why hadn't Chris been able to pray? "Lord," Chris whispered now, choking back tears, "I don't even deserve to talk to you. But I'm not asking for myself. It's for Bill. Please protect him. . . ."

An hour later, Chris found Bill at a gas station. "I was going to do it," Bill admitted, trembling. "I had the gun at the grave. But I just couldn't . . ."

"I prayed for you, man," Chris said.

"Thanks," Bill mumbled. "I guess it helped."

Praying for his friend in the hot spring sun marked the beginning of Chris's conversion experience. A few weeks later he visited his older brother, who was living in a Christian student group house on a West Coast university campus. Chris met self-confident and thoughtful young people who accepted him, despite his greasy doper's hair, black jeans and T-shirt, and childish provocation of his eyebrow ring.

They were working to build their lives, not screwing up their brains with speed, pot, and alcohol. But they did not exude the sanctimonious disdain of the "country club Christian" kids back home. "Living your faith doesn't mean you have to act better than anybody else," one of his brother's housemates told Chris.

Almost two years since Chris prayed so desperately for his friend in that thicket of loblolly pines, he is still struggling to complete his high school diploma, taking only one or two courses a semester. He no longer drinks, smokes tobacco or marijuana, or listens to death-haunted heavy metal rock. Chris has joined a church with an active youth program, where the younger kids respect him for his woodsman's skills. On camping trips, Chris talks to them frankly about drugs and alcohol.

Facing long odds, Chris plans to enter college, knowing full well it might take him ten years to earn a degree. By any psychological measure, he has broken free of depression. "I wouldn't say that I survived," Chris reflects. "God reached down and saved me."

Religion and Adolescent Mental Health: Donahue's Study

Chris Benfield's journey through those painfully stressful years is far from unique. The mental health profession is finally accepting the strong evidence that religion can protect young people from the severe distresses of contemporary adolescence.

In 1995, psychologists Michael J. Donahue and Peter L. Benson published what is probably the most thorough review of accumulated research on the relationship between religion and adolescent mental health.[19] The research they analyzed included "an unusually rich data set" drawn from several hundred thousand public school students in communities across the country. After screening this data for an unintended geographical bias toward the Middle West, Donahue and Benson scrutinized a representative sampling of 34,129 detailed questionnaires, designed to compare overall behavior and emotional adjustment with religious attitudes and practice.

They found that monthly or more frequent church attendance averaged around 50 percent of the sample. More than half of these young people stated that religion played an important part in their lives. "American adolescents are religious," the authors concluded, "and their average level of religiousness has not declined" in recent years.[20]

The researchers found that religion was "positively associated" with emotionally healthy values and socially accepted behavior, such as the tutoring or other volunteer work often organized by a religious congregation. Religious students were less likely to harbor suicidal thoughts or to make actual attempts on their lives. These religious students also showed significantly lower levels of drug and alcohol abuse, premature sexual involvement, and criminal delinquency. In other words, religion appeared to protect a highly representative sampling of young people from the negative effects of an increasingly stressful adolescence in America.

The authors of this important study recommend that future government and private initiatives meant to protect youth from substance abuse, violence, and the consequences of premature sexual activity include the participation of religious organizations. "Religion has some manifestly positive effects on behavior," they emphasized. "When it comes to a wide variety of at-risk behaviors that are concerns to people who work with youth, religion works; it should be allowed more space to do so."[21]

Chapter Six

Religion Offers Protection from Depression and Helps Those Afflicted to Recover Quickly

Depression in America

Last year [1998], the *Journal of the American Medical Association* reported dramatic findings on the "substantial growth in the number of depression visits" to physicians between 1985 and 1994, which almost doubled, from 10.99 million to 20.43 million annual consultations.[1] The study noted that new antidepressant medications, including Prozac, have replaced tranquilizers as the most commonly prescribed medication for emotional problems.[2]

The National Institute of Mental Health estimates that approximately 17.6 million Americans suffer depression each year, annually costing the nation up to $44 billion in treatment charges and lost wages.[3] Obviously, depression is a serious emotional disorder that is becoming increasingly common.

Like most illness, depression has a spectrum of severity, ranging from a transient but annoying emotional discomfort to a major, clinical condition. When people become severely depressed, they give up hope that their life will ever improve. They also often become nervous and irritable and lose interest in activities they once enjoyed. Depressed people can experience difficulty sleeping (or staying awake) or have trouble concentrating. They tend to withdraw from others. Usually they suffer the irrational, but agonizing, conviction that they are worthless. The anguish of depression can be so severe that many consider suicide, and about 15 percent of depressed people actually kill themselves.

Depression can also follow physical, emotional, and sexual abuse or other traumatic psychological shock, often striking when a person suffers the stress of a loss, such as the death of or separation from a loved one. But other forms of loss—losing a job, a financial setback, or failing health—can also trigger depression.

People inherit a certain genetic vulnerability to depression. But the entire complex of life experience can increase or decrease a person's susceptibility.

Many of the patients I've treated first became depressed because poor health undercut their independence and left them feeling socially isolated.[4] Some suffered physical discomfort—chronic pain, nausea, constipation, difficulty in breathing—or had mobility problems that made it difficult to even bathe and dress.

I think it's vital for people to understand that depression has major *physical health* consequences. Severe depression stemming from physical illness can exacerbate the disease and even provoke premature death. Chronic, unmitigated depression may itself be the root cause of many life-threatening diseases. In Chapter Eleven, we discuss the physiological pathways that link chronic stress with depression and serious physical illnesses such as cancer, cardiovascular disease, and immune system dysfunction.

But the good news is that people who enjoy religious faith appear better able to endure life's unavoidable hardships—running the gamut from a nasty boss to the death of a loved one—with what we aptly call "grace under pressure." They suffer depression like the rest of us, but they usually rebound quickly because their faith protects them from an emotionally wrenching sense of permanent isolation.

Rachel Cowan's Odyssey of Faith

Rabbi Rachel Cowan's journey through bereavement provides a good example of how faith and religious community help people rebound from depression following one of life's greatest emotional traumas, the premature death of a spouse.

In the late 1980s, Rachel Cowan and her husband Paul were entering a period of fulfillment. They had married during the civil rights movement of the turbulent 1960s. Paul became a respected staff writer for the *Village Voice* and wrote a critically acclaimed memoir tracing the spiritual meaning of his Jewish heritage, *An Orphan in History*.[5]

Paul had been raised in a prominent Jewish family that had turned its back on its roots. His grandparents had changed their name from Cohen to Cowan, which Paul grew up assuming was of Welsh origin. His family had embraced the dominant Christian culture, right down to celebrating Easter with a big ham dinner. It was not until Paul had graduated from Harvard and was working as a journalist that he began to explore what he called "cohesive, communal Judaism."

As his own religious commitment deepened, he began to encourage Rachel's curiosity about the faith. She had been raised in a traditional New England Unitarian family, but converted to Judaism in 1980. Rachel and Paul joined the effort to revitalize the once-thriving Ansched Chesed Temple on New York's Upper West Side. Four years later, Paul encouraged Rachel to begin rabbinical training at Hebrew Union College in New York.

In 1987, Rachel and Paul had been married twenty-two years; they had raised children, collaborated on books, and their bond of love was close. Their attributes complemented one another in such a way that each felt most complete as a person only when they were together.

Then one warm September night Paul became very sick. His joint pain, persistent fever, and extreme fatigue alarmed them both. Instead of waiting to see a doctor in the morning, Rachel took Paul to the emergency room of New York Hospital.

The initial lab tests seemed to take hours as Rachel paced anxiously in the crowded waiting room. Then a tired young doctor in wilted green scrubs appeared. "It looks like very bad news," he said, holding her hand. "We think Paul has leukemia."

Rachel's mind swirled with a dizzying sense of unreality. In her last year of the rabbinical seminary, she was studying grief counseling. "No . . . ," she muttered. "I'm the rabbi. I'm supposed to do this for someone else."

Within days, all possibility of mistaken diagnosis was ruled out, as was any confusion about what Rachel's role in this unfolding tragedy would be. Paul suffered a virulent and aggressive form of leukemia, a malignant cancer that attacks the body's complex blood-production system. Their normal world collapsed. Paul became a full-time passenger on the consultation-diagnosis-treatment treadmill that overwhelms so many gravely ill patients in our vast and complex heath care system. Rachel had to balance the demanding responsibilities of wife, mother, housekeeper, and editor of Paul's work-in-progress while trying to be his spiritual adviser.

Paul's treatment required long hospital stays away from friends and loved ones. Both he and Rachel found themselves increasingly isolated. After the initial weeks of denial, Rachel had to confront the fact that Paul was not going to experience a sudden and complete remission, as had an acquaintance of theirs, Rabbi Hirshel Jaffe, who had written eloquently of the spiritual aspects of his recovery in *Why Me? Why Anyone?*[6] When Rachel had read the book before Paul's diagnosis, she'd been overwhelmed by the prospect of becoming a rabbi and administering to the spiritual needs of people with life-threatening diseases. Now she faced this challenge with her beloved life partner, Paul.

Fighting her own anxious despair, Rachel realized it was her responsibility to create hope in Paul so that he would not be overwhelmed by depression, which she knew could undercut the effectiveness of his treatment. Spiritual hunger had been the main reason for Paul's return to Judaism. He had written that faith meant accepting the difficult realization that life is unpredictable, that God has given us "treasures and sorrows that none of us can foresee."

Rachel understood how much comfort the rich liturgy of the religion brought Paul. But she was not prepared for the spontaneous outpouring of support they both received from their synagogue and from Rachel's colleagues at Hebrew Union College.

Members of the Ansched Chesed congregation cooked kosher meals to tempt Paul's appetite, which had been eroded by chemotherapy. It was not unusual for Rachel to return to his hospital room and find people from the synagogue laughing and chatting with Paul as they encouraged him to nibble a few bites of knish.

When Sukkoth, the autumn Feast of Tabernacles, came, Paul was placed in a sealed isolation room because the disease had ravished his immune system. So Rabbi Nancy Flam had the students in her Hebrew class make colorful but sterile replicas of the boughs and fruits traditionally used to transform Jewish dining rooms into rustic harvest booths for the feast, and to then hang the streamers and cutouts above Paul's bed, softening the gleaming metal and beeping monitors so that this lonely corner of the isolation ward indeed became a sukkah ringing with laughter.

During the prayers, songs, and festive food, Rachel watched Paul put aside his burdensome preoccupation with his disease. Ironically, however, it was at these joyful moments, when Paul responded with his old warmth and innate optimism, that Rachel felt most intensely the cold, stabbing dread of impending loss. Her own isolation seemed to deepen, and with it the grip of depression tightened. There were times when she seemed suddenly drained of physical strength, torn by a fear so great that she was sure her knees would collapse and she would fall to the floor.

Then she suffered true spiritual anguish. While she was alone in prayer, crushing insights would intrude. *Why am I praying to You? Look what You have done to Paul, to me.* After each of these periods of despair, however, Rachel found the strength to pray again, strengthened by the faith that God had not chosen this illness to punish either her or Paul.

One of the most painful aspects of her emotional state was the mounting sense that Paul was slipping away from her emotionally as the physical disease progressed. They had always shared their intimate thoughts; now he was entering a territory she had never experienced. Rachel dreaded the idea that their bond of love would be stretched and broken even before Paul reached the end of his physical limits.

But religion offered the means to comfort both of them and to preserve their bond of intimacy.

One of the loneliest times came during Paul's preparation for a bone marrow transplant in a New England hospital. In this frightening experience, Paul lay alone beneath the chill, humming mass of a linear accelerator, undergoing total body radiation, which would kill his bone marrow—both malignant and healthy—so he could undergo the transplant. Rachel sat in the hall outside, forcing herself to read from the Psalms, trying to focus the timeless power of the Hebrew prayers on Paul's recovery.

When they wheeled Paul out, he was tired and anxious. "Could we think of a blessing about radiation?" he asked. "The only image I have is from nuclear bombs. I sure don't want to dwell on that."

Rachel's thoughts jumped through the important scriptural references she had learned in the seminary. With one hand holding Paul's, she leafed through her Bible. Then she came to the last chapter of Malachi, the final stanzas of the original Hebrew text. Here was the blessing she'd been searching for. "But for you who revere My name, the Sun of righteousness shall rise up with healing. . . ."

In the coming weeks, Rachel managed to find similar scriptural passages that brought them both a sense of inner peace. Sometimes she would mix scripture with snatches of the old civil rights songs—which themselves drew heavily on the Bible—and they would hold hands, singing softly.

Paul Cowan entered the terminal crisis of his illness just before the High Holiday of Rosh Hashanah, the festival of the Jewish New Year that brings the faithful spiritual renewal. As his death approached, Rachel was able to move beyond her depression and paralyzing anxiety. She saw that Paul was still able to appreciate the kindness of friends and loved ones. He could still enjoy the sunlight on the autumn foliage outside the hospital window, share a warm recollection from the past, even appreciate the aroma of food. *God*, Rachel realized, *is in the small details, the little things that happen each day.*

Rabbi Hirshel Jaffe helped the Cowans celebrate Rosh Hashanah in Paul's hospital room. When the last of the age-old prayers ended, Paul's eyes were shining with joy, and Rachel knew his spirits were soaring. Even though she faced the agony of grief, joining Paul in his final religious celebration filled her too with joy. Paul Cowan died during those holidays, at forty-eight.

After Paul's funeral service at the crowded Ansched Chesed Temple, Rachel returned to her rabbinical studies. She found herself surrounded by a loving community that allowed her to work through her grief by guiding it toward a religious context. Friends reminded her of comforting scriptural passages, including the verses in Deuteronomy in which the Lord tells the Hebrews that He has set before them "life and good, death and evil."

There is a choice, even in the face of death, Rachel saw. "I chose life." This marked the true beginning of her passage from depression and grief to optimistic faith. One of the greatest challenges a rabbi faces, she learned, is to help sick people repair their relationship with God. And Rachel recognized that she had only become fit for the task by passing through the trial of Paul's illness and death.

Rachel Cowan became a pioneer in the Jewish healing movement in North America. Her sense of loss is still profound, but she has endowed her bereavement with religious meaning. Every Sabbath evening at the lighting of the candles, she feels Paul's presence in her home. Rather than suffering an unending sense of loss, she experiences gratitude for the wonderful years they had together. "When you have religious faith," she notes, "you live with constant reminders of hope."

Faith and Bereavement

There are two aspects of Paul and Rachel Cowan's compelling story that I find especially germane to this book. First, neither had been raised a Jew, but both eventually found desperately needed emotional support in the richly spiritual beliefs, liturgy, and traditions of Judaism. Without the comfort of religion, I think, they both would have suffered major depression that could have blighted their last precious months together. And, although Rachel did not convert to Paul's faith until she was an adult, she found great solace in providing the support of this faith during his illness, a process psychologists call "religious helping."

But is their experience truly relevant to others? It would appear so. First, there is evidence suggesting that nonobservant Jews—like lapsed members of Christian denominations—are more prone to depression than their religious peers. Two related pioneering British studies published in the 1970s found that Jewish people suffering depression were significantly less religious than emotionally healthy Jews. One suggested explanation, of course, was that the faith and practice of Judaism may protect people from developing depression. One study even concluded that "loosening of communal bonds and/or weakening of religious behavior is of particular relevance to depression among Jews" when compared with the Protestant majority.[7]

Rachel Cowan and countless other bereaved men and women rebound from the depression of their loss by easing their grief through religious coping. Several studies of this emotionally healing process support the conclusion that religious faith mitigates the often crippling anguish unleashed when a loved one dies. A well-designed study of older widows and widowers attending southern California support groups found that people with deeply held personal ("intrinsic") faith had fewer depressive symptoms than their bereaved peers who reported that they felt their religious faith less intensely.

Research on Midwestern parents who'd lost young children to cancer and blood disorders revealed that the emotional comfort of religious faith helped most of them adjust to their loss. And, in an echo of Rachel Cowan's experience, many of these parents reported that their religious faith was actually strengthened by their loss.[8]

Adolescents who lose brothers or sisters are especially vulnerable to serious depression. But a study of bereaved Midwestern teenagers published in 1991 suggests that faith helps young people rebound from this depression. The teenagers in the study who found religion valuable were initially more depressed than their less religious peers, and suffered the common symptoms of intrusive images of their dead sibling, suicidal thoughts, and eating disorders. In contrast, the nonreligious teenagers reported emotional numbness and fear, among other depressive symptoms, immediately following the death of a brother or sister. But two years after the sibling's death, the religious adolescents had many fewer symptoms of depression than their nonreligious peers, most of whom still reported feeling depressed, being confused, and having trouble eating.[9]

The protective benefits of religious faith and membership in a congregation for bereaved people suggested in this research should obviously be studied more extensively. But I can confirm there is strong evidence that providing religious succor to others (one of Rachel Cowan's principal coping methods) aids vulnerable people in recovering from depression.

Faith and Coping

In 1997, I reported to the annual meeting of the American Psychiatric Association on research that my friend Kenneth I. Pargament of Bowling Green State University and I had conducted on the relationship between coping techniques and the mental health outcomes of older patients hospitalized with a variety of physical illnesses. We compared religious coping methods with nonreligious strategies among 577 men and women admitted to the Duke University Medical Center or to the Durham, North Carolina, Veterans Affairs Medical Center between January 1996 and April 1997.[10]

We defined religious coping as the use of religious beliefs and behaviors to prevent or alleviate the negative emotional consequences of stressful life circumstances and to facilitate problem solving.

Previous research had investigated religious coping very broadly, using one or two general questions. We wanted to be much more rigorous, and eventually identified twenty-one specific types of religious coping as well as eleven methods of nonreligious coping. We further separated religious coping into positive and negative behaviors.

To measure health outcomes we carefully assessed the patients' physical health, depressive symptoms, perceived quality of life, any personal growth they felt they'd achieved from the stressful experience of their illness, their level of cooperation during the interview process, and finally, whether they experienced spiritual growth from this stress.

Positive religious coping included a "reappraisal" of God as benevolent, attempting to collaborate with God, seeking a closer bond with God, and reaching out to clergy and church members for emotional support. We identified the final element of positive coping as "giving religious help to others." This included seeking out sicker patients and praying for them, offering spiritual help to them, and encouraging them spiritually.

Negative religious coping included believing that God was using illness to punish and that demonic forces were involved with poor health, pleading for direct divine intercession to cure a condition, or experiencing general spiritual discontent, all of which interfered with a sense of closeness to God. You'll recall that Rachel Cowan encountered this type of spiritual discontent when she found prayer fruitless, and even began to blame God for her husband's illness. Unfortunately, these negative patterns occur more frequently than most mental health workers realize.

After administering bedside interviews on both religious and nonreligious coping methods and charting the patients' faith practices with questions such as, "How often do you attend church or other religious meetings?" we assessed their mental health. This involved examination of memory and concentration, depressive symptoms, overall quality of life, stress-related growth, general cooperation, and spiritual growth. Finally, we measured the impact of the patients' illness on their religious faith, having them rate themselves on three statements: "I have grown closer to God," "I have grown closer to my church," and "I have grown spiritually."

We put the thousands of individual answers through a three-step linear regression statistical analysis which met the most rigorous standards of contemporary psychological research.

Almost 80 percent of our subjects rated their health as fair or poor, which suggested a high level of stress, so we weren't surprised to find that almost two-thirds of them showed symptoms of clinical depression.

The majority of the people in this study used such positive religious coping techniques as "seeking spiritual support" from clergy and church members, "active religious surrender" (choosing to trust completely in God and turn their problems over to him), and "religious purification," which involved prayers for forgiveness and atonement. Negative religious coping was much less frequent, but we did encounter people who blamed God for their illness or questioned God's power over their lives, and also people who were driven by stress into disagreements or squabbles with their clergy and church members.

The results of our analyses were intriguing. The higher the level of positive religious coping, the lower the level of depressive symptoms and the better the quality of life. In other words, those patients who used their religious faith in a positive manner experienced less depression and enjoyed a better overall emotional state (quality of life) than those who did not. The statistical analysis showed that this apparent protection from depression was not affected by the patients' age, sex, race, education, admitting hospital, or level of physical illness.

On the other hand, patients who resorted to negative religious coping showed higher levels of depression and poorer quality of life.

Some nonreligious coping methods such as denial, emotional "venting" (angry outbursts), or the use of alcohol or drugs were associated with both poorer physical and emotional health. But, while other seemingly positive nonspiritual coping techniques initially appeared related to better mental and physical health outcomes, their significance decreased under careful analysis. For example, using humor, actively designing coping strategies, and attempting to find good in the situation had little impact on physical or mental health. Only seeking emotional support from a close-knit circle of family or friends, and cultivating an attitude of acceptance, was associated with better emotional health.

In other words, religious coping techniques appear to provide the most good results.

We found the relationship between coping methods and personal and spiritual growth of particular interest. Of the twenty-one separate religious coping methods we examined, sixteen were positively and significantly associated with stress-related growth.

Religious Helping

Religious helping of others appeared to be a highly beneficial coping method related to better mental health. We found that older people who coped with their physical illness by reaching out to offer spiritual support and comfort to others were less likely to be depressed, experienced higher quality of life, showed high levels of stress-related personal growth, and were generally more cooperative. This finding was consistent with the growing body of research that suggests people who provide close friendship and emotional support to others enjoy improved well-being.[11] Certainly friendships involving sports and hobbies, child-rearing, cultural pursuits such as museum visits, and membership in clubs or groups offer such support. But it's interesting to note that faith communities often provide all these activities, with the added dimension of a spiritual bond.

Let's consider for a moment the people in this book who have given religious help and how this has protected them from stress or depression. For years, Walter Grounds was an energetic member of his church's annual religious pageants; Helen Koebert regularly helps in the religious training of preschool students; after Lorene Burns was diagnosed with Alzheimer's disease, her husband Paul devoted himself to helping others in spiritual need; Chris Benfield is now a youth worker in his church; and, of course, Rabbi Rachel Cowan actively promotes emotional healing within the traditions and liturgy of Judaism. Our data suggested that the emotionally protective aspects of religious helping transcend the type of cognitive distraction we often call "getting beyond your problems" by thinking of something else, perhaps a baseball game or a mindless thriller on HBO.

Religious helping provides an empowering sense of value and purpose that promotes inner tranquillity and eases emotional pain. Praying with and for another person is an act that is simultaneously intimate and dignified, which elevates a person above the unpleasant physical reality of his affliction or condition. Think of George Ortiz kneeling with Rick in that spartan storefront drug shelter in North Philadelphia, teaching him the healing words from Hebrews 13:5. "I will never leave you nor forsake you." That act of loving kindness did not miraculously transport the two men beyond the grim inner-city streets to prosperous happiness in the suburbs. But helping a virtually lost soul rise above the emotional hell of addiction strengthened George's own emotional state.

As I discuss my research with colleagues across the country, I encourage them to assess their patients' spiritual assets as well as their physical illness. A person may be bedridden, but able to read scripture to someone whose voice had been silenced by a stroke or a respirator. One of the most important findings of this research study is that we are multidimensional beings who have strength and resolve we can mobilize when our bodies are afflicted. And by mobilizing that strength and resolve to assist others spiritually, we help ourselves, both physically and emotionally.

Frank Kozoman's Journey out of Despair

There are times, of course, when physical disability strikes without warning and so severely that despair initially seems the most rational human response. But the story of Frank Kozoman shows us that depression does not have to smother emotional recovery.

On the cool Carolina Saturday afternoon of December 16, 1995, Frank Kozoman, then fifty-nine, climbed down the roof of his suburban home after stringing a web of Christmas lights. Kozoman was a muscular man determined to hold middle age at bay through regular exercise. He had left the security of academic engineering research to start his own analytical instrument company several years earlier.[12]

During the stress of a divorce and adapting to entreprenurial life, Kozoman had found comfort in his evangelical Protestant faith. He was a loyal member of the Christian Assembly Church, but tried to balance religion with the other demands of life and did not consider himself unusually devout.

As Frank stepped over the edge of the roof, his foot slipped off the aluminum extension ladder. He lurched down, his leg caught on the ladder. One moment he'd been on the roof, the next he was plunging backward, head down. Frank managed to lunge upward, an awkward midair sit-up that spared his head and neck. But he landed squarely on his lower back, a savage blow that numbed him from the hips down.

Two men working on the house next door rushed to his aid. Then

Susan, his wife of seven years, was suddenly standing above him. "Can you move your feet?" one of the workmen asked, his tone hushed and grave.

Frank strained, but his legs remained motionless on the grass, as if they belonged to someone else. *Maybe it's just shock*, he thought.

He managed to keep his optimism intact even as he was wheeled into surgery later that week. But when he emerged from anesthesia in the recovery room, a resident had the same somber expression as the workman in the yard had worn. "How long was I under?" Frank asked.

"Hours," the doctor replied. "We had to remove a lot of bone splinters from your spinal cord."

The resident's words stung like a whip. Frank raised his head and stared at the humps of his feet beneath the blanket, willing his legs to move. The realization was cold and sudden. *I'm paralyzed.*

Physical pain quickly replaced anguish. Fortunately, Frank had an intravenous morphine pump, electronically controlled to prevent overdose. Keeping himself heavily sedated, Frank was almost able to avoid the grim truth. But his doctors weaned him from narcotic pain medication when he entered the rehabilitation ward. Even though the rooms and corridors were cheerfully lighted, Frank saw the hospital in bleak shadows.

People from his church had spread a wide computer-printed banner, "Jesus Christ is Lord and He loves Frank Kozoman," above his bed. When Susan visited with Frank's grown son, Gene, they commented on the hopeful banner. Frank clenched his jaw to keep from lashing out angrily. But that night, alone in bed, he was overwhelmed with despair. He couldn't escape the image of Susan and Gene hiding their pity with polite conversation. Frank, who had come to treasure his independence, understood that he would henceforth always be dependent on people for his most mundane physical needs. That was simply not acceptable. He turned his face toward the wall and prayed from a center of misery much worse than his physical pain. *Why don't you just end it now?* he asked God, as if addressing an impersonal bureaucrat.

Frank built a shell of pain and irritability around his body, focusing his depression on the caregivers. He made a token effort at following the physical therapists' instructions. But inside he was seething, beginning to focus on one goal: ending his life. During this dark period, he spoke to Gene on the telephone. "I want you to bring over that big forty-four pistol of yours," Frank said in a calm tone. "But I'll just need one bullet."

His son gasped, then snapped back, "Dad, you can just go to hell. If you work hard, you'll be up again. You can make a life if you want to."

"Maybe I don't want to," Frank answered.

While Frank was still burdened with pain and churning with depression, a member of his congregation, retired University of North Carolina psychiatry professor Dr. Harry Derr, came to the hospital to visit. Derr took Frank's hand and almost forced him to join in prayer. Then Derr began to discuss Frank's condition in candid and uncompromising detail. Finally, Derr accurately described the classical symptoms of depression Frank was suffering. "You think you're being unfairly punished," Derr said. "You believe no one else has ever been in your position. But I want you to remember one thing: There is life on the other side of this and you will adjust to it."

Frank had turned his face away from Derr and stared at the annoying electronic squiggles on the monitors that charted the painfully tedious functions of his crippled body. He did not want to adjust to this empty existence. Yet here was Harry Derr, able to walk wherever he wanted, use a toilet like a normal person, and stand in a shower, burdening Frank with these platitudes.

"If I could get up," Frank growled, "I'd smack you one."

"I'll be back tomorrow," Derr replied. "Remember what I told you. God bless you."

Derr returned every day, bringing prayer and his unvarnished assessment of Frank's depression. One day he commented on an array of get-well cards the kids in Sunday school had painted. " 'We're praying for you, Mr. Kozoman,' " Derr read. " 'Get well soon.' What do you think of that?"

Frank studied the children's work. "I suppose their teachers made them do it" was all he said.

"But they *are* praying for you," Derr insisted.

"I suppose so." Frank shrugged.

"If they can," Derr said, "why can't you?"

Frank pondered the question for hours after Derr left. When the shift changed that afternoon, a nurse also noticed the cards. "Mr. Kozoman," she asked, "do you mind if some of us pray for you?"

"I guess not," Frank mumbled, then fully considered her question. Strangers here at the hospital who had seemed so emotionally detached were willing to spend time praying for him. How could he refuse them?

Before his accident, Frank had been studying Hebrews with his meticulous attention to detail. Now his eye fell to Chapter 11, Verse 6: "And without faith it is impossible to please Him, for he who comes to God must believe that He is, and that He is a rewarder of those who seek Him."

Frank now spent hours each day carefully analyzing biblical passages. He detected a pattern in chapter after chapter: God repeatedly tested people's faith through painful trial, only to strengthen them. That was the "other side" that Harry Derr had described.

While Frank was embarked on this spiritual journey, he became increasingly aware of the loving presence of his church congregation, which he hadn't noticed during the initial cloud of depression. People dropped in before work to pray with Frank. Couples came in the afternoon with homemade pot roast or foil-wrapped dishes of chicken and dumplings.

Church member Don Casner arrived early on a Wednesday and proposed to work for a year without salary to keep Frank's business going. Another member of the congregation offered him an interest-free loan to preserve Frank's cash-flow business during this "temporary" medical crisis. Frank understood for the first time since the accident that he could in fact continue to sell scientific instruments from a wheelchair. As Harry Derr had predicted, life would continue, *if* Frank did not reject it.

I visited Frank just before he was scheduled for discharge. Unlike so many other physically ill or disabled religious people I had seen in my career, Frank showed no obvious signs of depression. His expression was animated, his thoughts clear, and his manner optimistic. He lifted his well-thumbed Bible. "My church and my faith are helping me through this, Doctor," he said.

So far, so good, I thought, knowing the real test of his psychological recovery would come when he returned home and had to confront the immutable daily burden of his disability in the normal world of the physically able.

But once more, the congregation rallied to Frank's side. Frank and Susan's old frame house was spacious but, with the bathroom up a flight of stairs, impractical for someone in a wheelchair. David Crabtree, a general contractor, organized other craftsmen from the church. Less than a month after Frank returned home, Crabtree and his volunteers had donated more than two hundred man-hours to convert a laundry into a large, fully furnished handicapped bathroom, charging the Kozomans only the wholesale cost of the major fixtures.

Later, when the Kozomans prepared to move into their new single-floor home, church members volunteered to paint the old house and help with the drudgery of packing. Frank hardly knew many of these volunteers, yet they cheerfully packed books and wrapped dishes with the same care they would have given their own possessions. It was during this move that he saw the true nature of his relationship to this congregation. They were not helping out of pity, but from love. He recognized a sincere bond uniting the members of this church that was, in many ways, closer than links connecting brothers and sisters in the widely dispersed families so prevalent in America today. And, like Khalita Jones and Rachel Cowan, Frank felt his need to respond to this love in a positive manner. He simply could not turn away from these people and surrender to the depression that was always haunting the edges of his mind.

Today Frank and Susan run their successful and expanding business from their new home. Like all self-employed people, they confront stress and uncertainty. And Frank also struggles with terrible complications of his injury. Twice since the accident he has undergone surgery on his spine and has been forced to endure agonizing weeks of complete immobility, lying supine on a fluid-filled bed.

There were long days and interminable nights during these recoveries when emotional darkness threatened to smother Frank once more. However, he has learned to fight this incipient depression through prayer and scriptural study. Frank believes that God is continually present in his life, that in an inexplicable way the accident, in which

Frank escaped a fatal neck or head injury by inches, has given him an unexpected opportunity to explore his faith.

"All of this has been a test," Frank reflects. "God has provided me the strength to endure. And each day He offers me a little bit more of the wisdom I need to understand."

Religion and Depression in Later Life

Frank Kozoman encountered disabilities earlier in life than most of us. But many elderly people hospitalized with the debilitating conditions common in later life must also confront depression. With a specialty in geriatric psychiatry, I recognize that coping with this type of depression will inevitably become a major health policy concern as our population ages and cost containment emerges as *the* crucial health care issue. Remember, depression undercuts people's ability to cooperate with medical treatment as well as their will to survive. As larger numbers of elderly people become depressed, they will need more care in hospitals and residential facilities. There's a danger that the system might be strained beyond its limits.

But the medical profession has not yet established practical clinical guidelines to incorporate patients' spirituality into the struggle against depression. I believe, however, that religious faith can become a cost-effective complement to psychotherapy and medication in this effort.

The desire to explore this exciting medical frontier led me to direct an ongoing series of research studies at Duke University on the relationship between religious faith and recovery from depression among people suffering physical illness.

The First Duke University Study on Depression and Religion: Men over Sixty-five

In one of the first major investigations I led at Duke, my team studied the level and effectiveness of religious coping among 850 men over sixty-five who were admitted to the medical and neurological services of a Veterans Administration hospital between September 1987 and January 1989.[13] They came from throughout the southern Mid-Atlantic region and represented a typical cross section of their peers, and had medical diagnoses of cancer and gastrointestinal, neurological, respiratory, renal, and cardiac diseases.

We screened them for symptoms of depression using standard diagnostic tests (the Geriatric Depression Scale and the Hamilton Depression Scale). There were indications that the degree and frequency of depression would fall into predictable patterns, including personal and family histories of psychiatric illness, poor physical health, and little social support.

What we had not predicted, however, was the level at which these men used their religious faith as a buffer against depression. When we asked them an open-ended question about how they coped with their physical illness or disability, 20 percent spontaneously replied that religion was their primary tactic. This involved trusting in God, praying, reading scripture or inspirational literature, following religious broadcasts, attending church services, and receiving emotional support from the clergy or members of their congregations. More than half of all the patients considered themselves very religious, and 21 percent listed religion as being "the most important thing that keeps me going."

When our data were put through statistical analyses, we found that the more a patient relied on religion, the lower his level of depressive symptoms. Further, we discovered that this apparent protective benefit of religion was stronger among men with more severe physical disability.

The religious patients told us that their strong personal belief and faith in God and their relationships to their church congregations gave them great comfort and a feeling of peace.

In analyzing religious coping by denomination, we discovered evidence that members of conservative, black, or fundamentalist/evangelical Protestant groups appeared to rely most on their religious faith to help them cope with health problems. The men who relied on religious coping also reported high levels of social contact and very low levels of alcohol use, which suggests that they had more support from other persons and thus had less of a need to cope with health problems by turning to alcohol. This type of personal bolstering reminded me of my earlier research in the Midwest, where more than half of the older patients I studied said that nearly all their closest friends came from their church congregations.

Our study also found that the more functionally disabled a man was, the greater the benefits he received from religious coping (in terms of being protected from depression). I think this is an important element in the apparent protective benefit of a strong personal faith and membership in a faith community. Consider the emotional impact of spontaneous loving support on gravely ill or disabled people such as Paul Cowan and Frank Kozoman.

Again, it seems plausible that personal religious faith and worship with others allow people to overcome feelings of helplessness and give meaning and a sense of control to those struggling with physical illness. It's worth repeating that depressed people are often consumed by feelings of hopelessness in their lives, which devout religious faith and practice help to combat.

The Duke University Study on Depression and Religion: Men and Women over Sixty

My Duke University research team has recently investigated the role of deep personal (intrinsic) faith as a factor in recovery from depression among older people hospitalized for physical illness. Between November 1993 and March 1996, we screened men and women patients over age sixty who were admitted to the general medicine, cardiology, and neurology services of Duke University Medical Center. Again we used standard diagnostic tests and personal interviews. This initial testing helped us identify eighty-seven patients with clinically significant depressive disorders.[14]

We then carefully assessed their intrinsic, or personal, religiosity with ten questions measuring the extent to which their faith in God was the main driving force in their lives—the primary motivating factor that affected all their decisions and habits. This was in contrast to "extrinsic" religiosity, where religion is used as a means to another end—such as social or economic prestige—rather than stemming from within the person, an end in itself. Finally, they answered detailed questions about the social support they received from family, friends, and community services.

After the depressed patients were released from the hospital, we followed up with a series of telephone interviews to discover who among them would recover from depression, how long it would take, and whether intrinsic religious faith was an important factor in this recovery.

Our results were quite interesting. Among the eighty-seven patients in the final study group, fifty had major depression and thirty-seven had significant, but less severe depression. Slightly more than half recovered from the depression in the year following their discharge from the hospital. Among those who "remitted" (got better), the median time for remission from depression was thirty weeks, with a range of one to fifty weeks.

After examining twenty-eight different variables, including quality of life, family history of psychiatric disorders, severity of physical illness and change in severity over time, social support, and treatment with antidepressants, we learned that intrinsic religiosity was one of the most important factors in speed of recovery. The higher a person's intrinsic religiosity, the faster he or she recovered from depression.

To our knowledge, this is the first "prospective" investigation (a research study that follows patients over time) to examine the effects of religiosity on speed of recovery from clinically significant depressive disorder. Our data showed that for every ten-point increase on the intrinsic religiosity score, there was a 70 percent increase in speed of recovery.

Was this just a random association? I certainly do not think so, given the similarity in findings with our earlier study of 850 hospitalized veterans, which convincingly demonstrated that the higher the level of religious coping, the lower the number of depressive symptoms.

In the second study, we selected patients who had been diagnosed with significant clinical depression. We asked these depressed patients at the beginning of the second Duke study what *they* thought enabled them to cope with the stress of their physical illness and other depressing elements of their lives. One-third spontaneously gave religious responses, such as "God," "The Lord," "My faith," or "Prayer."

In my discussing the findings of these studies with other medical professionals, several major implications occurred to me. First, most physicians and psychologists still do not recognize the healing potential of religious faith in people's lives. Clinicians treating people in hospitals emphasize the scientific (and often impersonal) aspects of therapy. But these same doctors, nurses, and psychologists play a role in controlling patients' access to chaplains, religious reading material and broadcasts, and hospital worship services. If health care professionals don't begin to recognize the power of religious faith to help people recover from depression, I believe a major healing resource will be wasted.

One of the most important lessons of the Duke research is that an active religious life can both shield people from depression and reduce its toll in terms of physical health. And, as we shall discuss in much greater detail later, significant depression can trigger the onset of physical illness by negatively influencing the cardiovascular and immune systems, which can lead to heart disease, stroke, and possibly cancer. But recovery from depression with the help of religion can boost people's participation in treatment and motivate them toward recovery. This is especially true in major illnesses of the elderly such as strokes and fractures due to osteoporosis.

Bill Maceri's Expression of Faith

Until recently, a diagnosis of HIV or AIDS was tantamount to a death sentence, as potentially depressing as learning you have terminal cancer. Countless thousands of AIDS patients have had to contend with major depression as well as their debilitating illness. And, even though the new combinations of anti-retroviral agents and protease inhibitor medications have brought remission to many people struggling with AIDS, depression often continues to haunt them.

Depression is a complication of the disease that presents problems beyond the pain of emotional anguish. The damage chronic depression can do to the immune system, which AIDS badly weakens, has been documented.[15]

Certainly people with AIDS could benefit from the healing power of faith and the support of a religious congregation in their recovery from depression. Unfortunately, many people infected with the AIDS virus are gay men or intravenous drug users (and their sexual partners) whose lifestyles have evoked at best an ambivalent response from religious communities. A few vociferous religious leaders have proclaimed the disease divine retribution for immorality, which has further alienated gay men with AIDS from churches and synagogues. As the story of Bill Maceri illustrates, however, a diagnosis of AIDS does not necessarily prevent a person from drawing strength and comfort from spiritual faith to battle depression.

Bill, now thirty-nine, was working as an actor and dancer in Berlin when he was diagnosed with HIV ten years ago. Homosexuality bore no stigma in the German artistic milieu Bill had lived in for years. Raised in a conventional Roman Catholic family in suburban Detroit, Bill had opted for the "hassle-free" life of an expatriate.

But two years after his diagnosis with HIV, Bill began to become symptomatic. Bouts of exhaustion undercut his athletic ability as a dancer. One evening he stumbled offstage after a performance, exhausted, and realized he just couldn't physically do this anymore and it would probably be better to return to America, where he could find a more familiar support system.

Once in New York, Bill decided to resume his original discipline of the visual arts because it was less physically demanding. But the relentless progression of the illness made it difficult for him to earn a living. He soon became emotionally and socially isolated, living in a studio in the blighted Bedford-Stuyvesant district of Brooklyn.

As the fever of opportunistic infections common to AIDS victims persisted, Bill's emotional perspective became somber. Some days, virtually drained by gastrointestinal infection, Bill would lay shivering in his isolated studio, listening to the occasional warble of police sirens on the streets below. He remembered the intellectually stimulating life he'd known in the tolerant enclave in West Berlin during the 1980s. He missed Europe.

It was at this time that Bill began to exercise his spiritual inclinations. Unlike many gay men with AIDS, Bill had maintained close relations with his family. He realized that it was his father's deep Catholic faith in God's unbroken love for all of creation that had preserved the family's bond.

Bill was able to intensify the unquestioning faith of his childhood, while his belief in the Christian Trinity and the Virgin Mother as the ultimate source of healing grace grew stronger. As HIV continued to spread in his body, he recalled prayer, meditations, and other spiritual practices learned through various theater and self-awareness workshops while living in Berlin, New Mexico, and Chicago. He grew to rely on a combination of Christian prayer and less traditional meditation to battle the encroaching darkness of depression.

Above all, it was a sense of peace that came from prayer that allowed Bill to overcome the anguished sense of worthlessness that plagues so many people with depression. One morning Bill awoke in his Brooklyn studio and decided there was more to life than this self-imposed banishment. "I realized that I did not have to live this way if I were self-empowered."

He was already struggling back from depression through the discipline of prayerful meditation when the new "cocktail" of AIDS medications became available. Bill's physical health rebounded with this treatment regimen. He found a rewarding job as an artist at an interior design studio and moved into a supportive new circle of friends.

The specter of AIDS and premature death never completely disappeared. Bill discovered, however, that he could successfully overcome anxiety and the smothering sensation of futility through the spiritual practices that had strengthened during the years of his illness. Beyond relief from the pain of depression, Bill Maceri has also begun to experience the tangible presence of spirituality working in his life.

"Once I decided to open my spiritual eyes," Bill says, "I began to receive a series of blessings."

Bill cites his improved physical health, his intensifying faith, his job,
his loving family, his outlets to exhibit art, and the support he receives
from his friends.

The terrible image of a painful and isolated death no longer tortures
Bill. He believes deeply that God will not abandon him. "I feel very
close to God, very supported," Bill says, describing his present outlook.

The Yale Study: AIDS and Religious Faith

Bill Maceri's recovery from the depression associated with AIDS is not
unique. A recent study led by researchers at Yale University School of
Medicine investigated the connection between religious faith and fear
of death among AIDS patients.[16] Dr. Lauris C. Kaldjian led the team
that surveyed the patients about their underlying fear of death, end-of-
life decisions (including resuscitation), guilt over HIV infection, and
religious faith.

About a third of the patients surveyed reported a fear of death;
around half of them expressed guilt about their HIV infection (which
often stemmed from using contaminated needles during drug abuse);
and more than a quarter believed their disease was some form of punishment for their lifestyle.

But when the patients' religious faith was factored in, the researchers found that fear of death was less prevalent among those who
read the Bible frequently, regularly attended church, or said that God
was very meaningful in their lives. The AIDS patients who believed in
God's forgiveness displayed less anxiety in discussing resuscitation and
other end-of-life considerations.

The Yale researchers noted, "Belief in a God who forgives and comforts may signify an ability to accept HIV infection or premature
death." Commenting on the study, Dr. David B. Larson, president of
the National Institute for Healthcare Research, observed, "A disease

like AIDS often creates a spiritual crisis for the patient through feelings of guilt and the belief that God is punishing the patient. This study shows that a strong religious commitment and belief in a forgiving God can help alleviate this crisis."

I certainly concur. Release from this "spiritual crisis" is often the type of faith-based recovery from depression that provides previously anguished people like Bill Maceri a sense of inner peace.

Shelly Cole's Battle with Depression

Tragically, people suffering mental illness are often stigmatized even more cruelly than AIDS patients. But Shelly Cole's amazing recovery from severe depression illustrates the healing potential of religious faith.

Shelly's account of her childhood and troubled adult life reminds me of a textbook case study on the root causes and crippling effects of serious depressive illness.

Now thirty-five, Shelly has suffered mental illness most of her life. Her troubles began as a young child in the Midwest when she was repeatedly sexually abused. She was violently raped at age sixteen and experienced the classic symptoms of post-traumatic shock, including emotional isolation and suicidal thoughts.

Shelly's emotional condition prevented her from completing a music degree at the University of North Carolina. As often happens to such abuse victims, Shelly unconsciously sought relief by marrying an emotionally distant and abusive person. She reports that her first husband's violence reached the point where he often threatened her with a .38-caliber revolver. But it is significant that Shelly's response to these savage assaults sprang from suicidal depression. "Why don't you go ahead and pull the trigger?" she once told her husband. "That would put us both out of our misery."

Shelly did manage to rebound well enough in the mid-1980s to recognize the danger of this relationship and was able to divorce the man and win custody of their daughter. But she was merely repressing deeper emotional wounds that had been inflicted on her in childhood.

She married her second husband impulsively after a brief courtship, again indicative of a fundamental insecurity related to her emotional illness. They had two children and lived an uneasy but financially stable life for several years. However, basic incompatibility and Shelly's underlying emotional illness eventually sparked serious friction in the marriage.

Faced with another divorce, she suffered a psychotic break in January 1995. One afternoon, when her children were on their way home from school, Shelly was seized by an overpowering compulsion, which possessed its own bizarre logic from the perspective of her depression. She loaded her husband's shotgun with buckshot and sat calmly in the living room, listening for the school bus. Her plan was cruelly simple: She would lead the children to the backyard, then shoot them, saving the last round of buckshot for herself. This act would "save" the children from the pain of losing their mother, put an end to her own misery, and spare her husband the burden of raising children alone.

Fortunately, she called her therapist, not ostensibly to seek help, but to say good-bye. "Thank you for all you've done for me," Shelly said. "I finally found an answer to my problems."

"Just let me put you on hold for a second," the therapist replied. While Shelly was holding, the other woman called 911. Heavily armed officers surrounded Shelly's home in rural Person County, North Carolina. Dennis Oakley, the local sheriff, bravely coaxed Shelly to the porch and talked her into handing over the shotgun.

Shelly was diagnosed with severe depression, suicidal tendencies, a borderline personality disorder, and multiple personality disorder, a typical pattern of emotional illness for the survivor of severe childhood abuse. For the next year, Shelly was hospitalized. As often happens in these seemingly intractable cases, her physicians prescribed increasing dosages of antidepressant and antipsychotic medications, including Effexor, Neurontin, and Librium, again with little apparent effect.

Then, ten months into her hospitalization, she was granted a weekend pass to accompany her sister, Kari, to a religious retreat for women. Shelly's experience with religion throughout her years of suffering had been unsatisfactory. As a disturbed child enduring abuse, one of her prayers had been, "Lord, just let me go to sleep and die."

At the retreat, she found herself standing before a group of neatly dressed, middle-class women, suddenly relating details of the wrenching traumas she'd experienced. Then Shelly saw a woman sitting alone at the rear of the room, her face rigid and distraught. As Shelly spoke, the woman covered her eyes, and tears spilled around her clenched fingers. Shelly had a sudden insight: *The Lord has brought me here to help this poor soul who has not yet found her voice.*

Shelly uttered an optimistic statement that she suddenly felt with absolute conviction. "No matter where you have been," she said, gazing at the suffering woman, who stared back through her tears, "there is always hope."

At the coffee that followed these testimonies, Shelly searched in vain for the woman. But it didn't matter whether she ever spoke to her again, Shelly realized. God had given her insight into the purpose of her lifelong pain. *I can help others.*

For the first time in her life, Shelly understood that there was an infinitely stronger power in the universe than her crushing fears and compulsions. A few weeks later she attended a healing service with her sister and experienced a rush of joyful optimism, a hopefulness that she had never before felt.

The hospital staff was amazed when Shelly's symptoms disappeared during the weeks following these religious experiences. She was released in January 1996. Later, her psychiatrist cautioned Shelly against cutting back too quickly on the powerful combination of medications.

"Doctor," Shelly told him, "I really am fine now and don't need all these pills. God didn't bring me this far to drop me on my face."

The doctor was duly skeptical; sudden withdrawal of these medications could be emotionally and physically dangerous.

But Shelly suffered absolutely no complications from withdrawal. Instead of tapering off, she quit "cold turkey" and began to substitute long meditative prayer and scriptural reading for the drugs.

Shelly Cole's religious conversion was similar in some ways to Rick's faith-based break with heroin. Shelly is firmly convinced that the Lord

has cured her of chronic mental illness. She feels a deep sense of fulfillment through sharing her faith with others and participating in regular
worship. In 1998, Shelly's church presented her its annual award as the
most active volunteer helper in the church.

As a psychiatrist who has treated people with serious depression, I
have no easy scientific explanation for Shelly's dramatic recovery. Unfortunately, there has not been much research on the therapeutic value
of such religious conversion. One study published in 1978, however,
indicates that this type of profound religious experience is associated
with significant reduction in symptoms of anxiety, depression, suicidal
thoughts, and related substance abuse.[17]

Although I would not suggest that any person should suddenly stop
his or her psychiatric medications, in view of Shelly Cole's recovery
from depression, I would certainly recommend that researchers consider investigating the full dimensions of the healing effect of profound
religious conversion experiences.

We will now examine the intriguing and growing body of evidence
that faith may provide equally dramatic benefits to the physical health
of religious people.

Chapter Seven

✳

Religious People Live Longer, Healthier Lives

Our Quest for Longevity

As my Baby Boom generation reluctantly enters middle age, the issue of longevity is becoming something of a national obsession. All you have to do is scan the health section of your local bookstore to find a cluster of new titles promising the secrets of staying alive, physically healthy, mentally acute, and even sexually active until you're a hundred. Are these claims just hyperbole aimed at a hedonistic generation that's been too spoiled to surrender the pleasures of youth and submit to the natural slings and arrows of aging? Probably.

But there is a solid and growing body of research showing that religiously active people may be both physically healthier into later life and actually living longer than their nonreligious counterparts. We've already seen evidence suggesting three explanations for this health and longevity among people with religious faith. First, religious people are more likely to have healthier lifestyles and avoid self-destructive behaviors than the nonreligious. Second, members of religious congregations often have their illnesses diagnosed earlier, are encouraged to seek better medical care, and are more compliant about medical treatment than the nonreligious. This is partially due to greater personal contact with concerned friends within a congregation. And the third reason religious people might enjoy greater health and longevity is that they are protected from the physical illnesses triggered by stress and depression.

A Long, Healthy Life

Many people I know have conflicting feelings about old age and longevity. On the one hand we wistfully read accounts of Biblical patriarchs such as Methuselah living for centuries; then we consider our own grandparents' life spans, which probably extended just into their seventies before failing health closed in. Certainly, most of us wish to live long, *healthy* lives. But we definitely don't want our older years to be a time of chronic illness and emotional isolation. Indeed, a recent survey by the U.S. Alliance of Aging Research found that 65 percent of Americans are deeply worried about "living for many years in a nursing home because of physical frailty or long-term illness."

Clearly, many of us fear that improving longevity will inevitably bring a declining quality of life, ending with painful disability and dependence. But there is nothing inevitable about this grim scenario. Medical science now has the means to detect early and treat successfully many of the disabling and life-threatening illnesses of people's later years. And research has shown that older people with positive outlooks and an overall sense of life satisfaction are less prone to depression and better able to overcome the discomforts and physical limitations that accumulate as we age.

With this in mind, ask yourself a couple of simple questions: What are the spiritual or religious lives of your optimistic and satisfied older friends and acquaintances? Are these people also healthy and reasonably active?

I'm confident that many of the lively and optimistic elderly around you draw emotional comfort and encouragement from their religious faith and religious involvement, as do all the healthy and energetic older men and women we've met in this book. To a person, they see their mature years as an opportunity for spiritual growth, a time of fulfillment, not limitation.

But I don't mean to imply that faith miraculously protects us from every illness. Religion is not a fountain of youth. Medical science now understands a great deal about the aging process at the cellular and even the molecular level; no gerontologist would suggest that anyone—even the most devout and religiously active—will advance beyond the eighth decade of life without some reduction in physical function. Religious people experience the same problems of arthritic joint deterioration, weakening eyesight, diminished respiratory capacity, and urinary difficulties as everyone else.

Remember, however, the distinction I made earlier between healing and cure. Faith gives people the inner strength and resolve needed to transcend the inescapable physical difficulties of aging and provides the emotional resiliency that is a key component in longevity.

Let's take another brief look at the contribution this emotional strength provides in the lives of older religious people who have shared their stories with us.

The Faithful Elderly

Marguerite and Walter Grounds have each included prayer in their daily lives for as long as they can remember. They experience a direct, personal connection with God. This helped sustain Walter during his impoverished childhood and also when the Groundses' daughter Janet was a helpless polio victim in an iron lung in Miami in 1949.

Such deeply felt faith includes elements of humility in the almost tangible presence of the Almighty and profound gratitude for the existence of a loving God who answers sincere prayers. When I did my early research on death anxiety among the religious elderly, I was impressed by the description of afterlife many offered spontaneously. They often described dying as "going home," or "joining" the Lord. Marguerite and Walter Grounds share such comforting faith. Their trust in God's providence allows them to overcome the inevitable physical afflictions of old age and preserve their optimism. In turn, this positive outlook and sense of well-being protects them from the stress of emotional isolation and depression that could undercut their physical health.

I think it's quite appropriate that clergy and sociologists now routinely use the term "faith community" to describe a religious congregation. The Groundses' close bond to the people of Cheek Height Baptist Church is a daily reminder that their lives have value. Sadly, this level of comforting social support is lacking in the lives of many elderly people in our increasingly mobile society. Often today, the people in a family are separated geographically or through divorce and remarriage from their children and grandchildren. The loneliness of such estrangement can be harshly painful to the elderly. All of us long for a sense of community, a need that does not diminish with age. Even though Marguerite Grounds's health problems have recently prevented her from attending church service, her congregation never ceases reminding her of their loving concern.

The importance of such a communal bond on health and mortality is hard to exaggerate. You'll recall that we discussed a pioneering study that found greater marital stability and well-being among religious kibbutzim dwellers in Israel compared with their secular peers. That large, multiyear research investigation also revealed higher overall mortality among the secular group. But this difference in death rates was most dramatic among people age seventy-five and older. During the sixteen years of the study, thirty-three of these elderly members of secular kibbutzim died, compared with only three of their religious counterparts. The researchers concluded there was a significant "protective effect of religious observance" at work among the observant. I also believe that membership in a close-knit family of the faithful contributes to such enhanced survival in subtle ways that science has only begun to measure.

Paul Burns, whose beloved wife Lorene was slowly taken from him by Alzheimer's disease, was especially vulnerable to stressful isolation when he moved to North Carolina. He had left his home community and church of almost fifty years and had no family or former professional colleagues in his new home. But virtually from the moment Paul joined the First Baptist Church, the congregation rallied around both him and Lorene. The greatest contribution the church members made to Paul's well-being might have been their unspoken assurance that he was a valuable member of their faith community.

Keep in mind that Paul Burns enjoyed the challenge of responsibility his entire adult life. He and Lorene had continued meeting substantive challenges in their ambitious colonial-home development after Paul retired. But when he found himself uprooted, Paul faced a potentially serious threat to his sense of self-worth, which is common among elderly retired men removed from their communities. Once again, however, the spiritual bond of membership in a congregation overcame isolation. To Paul Burns, the love these "new friends" gave to both Lorene and him was a true "blessing." This provided Paul the strength to reach beyond his own emotional pain and expand his perspective to search out others in need. I have no doubt that this spiritual growth, even coming late in life as it did, played a key role in Paul's continued emotional and physical health.

Scientific Evidence Connecting Faith and Longevity

Again, the stories of the Groundses and the Burnses are heartening, but they are what scientists correctly call anecdotal evidence. By themselves, such personal accounts do not scientifically prove that religion enriches and prolongs the lives of elderly people. For that we must rely on structured research studies that employ rigorous statistical analysis.

But there is a growing body of research evidence indicating a connection between social support (from group or community membership) and better physical health and improved longevity. Group membership often means belonging to a religious congregation and regularly attending services. A number of recent studies have also suggested a link between attendance at religious services and greater well-being, less depression and anxiety, less substance abuse, fewer suicides, better cardiovascular health, and longer survival. In fact, there is intriguing evidence that frequency of attendance at church or synagogue is an important independent—and largely unexplained—element in reducing death risk among average people.

*

The Strawbridge Study: Religion and Long Life

In the largest and best-designed study, William J. Strawbridge, Ph.D., and other California researchers examined the relationship between religious service attendance patterns and mortality of 5,286 people aged twenty-one to sixty-five in Alameda County between 1965 and 1994.[1] This landmark research, following as it did such a large group for such a long period of time, was so unique and was regarded as having such a high statistical reliability that it attracted major attention when it was published in the *American Journal of Public Health* in June 1997. The investigators carefully analyzed a volume of data collected through questionnaires at four intervals during the course of the long study. The main goal of the project was to analyze any long-term connection between attendance at religious service and reduced death risk, and the researchers hoped to determine if this apparent link could be explained principally by better health practices and closer social ties among frequent attenders.

Their major findings drew a fascinating picture of those people who seemed to derive the most overall health benefits from their religious involvement. People who attended religious services at least once a week, Strawbridge's team determined, were more likely to be women than men. Blacks tended to be more religiously involved than whites. As a group, frequent attenders had *more* health problems impairing their mobility than average, but also had higher levels of close family and social contacts and were more likely to be members of three or more community or neighborhood organizations. Frequent attendees also smoked and drank alcohol at much lower levels than their less religiously active peers.

One of the researchers' most significant findings when they measured mortality in the entire group was that the hazard of dying during the years of the study for the frequent religious service attenders was 36 *percent less* than for people who attended services less than once a week. Careful analysis of the data showed that some of this protection probably derived from the close family ties and friendships these people enjoyed and from their better health practices.

Even when these important factors were considered, however, the more religiously involved people *still* had an overall *23 percent reduced risk of dying between 1965 and 1994.*

The team also found an interesting gender difference. The observed connection between frequent attendance and reduced mortality was stronger among women than men, results similar to earlier, more limited research. Why was this so? Strawbridge and his colleagues noted that women generally attend religious services more frequently than men and have often shown stronger religious commitment. The researchers surmised that more women than men use religion to cope with life stress, which has been confirmed in other studies. And, based on earlier research, the Strawbridge study noted: "There is also evidence that religious involvement has stronger protective associations for disability and depression among older women than among older men." Because there's a higher proportion of older women who have lost their mates than men who have lost theirs, the team added, religious involvement may fill otherwise unmet needs for companionship.

Research that I have led at Duke also suggests that religion is more important for women because of their traditionally more limited involvement in activities that bring them social recognition and prestige outside the home. Becoming active in a congregation often gives a woman a vital sense of purpose, self-esteem, and satisfaction that fulfills them more deeply than the prestige of career achievement that so many men seek to the exclusion of their spiritual lives. And this type of religious satisfaction helps bolster a positive outlook, which in turn can lead to better health practices, a sense of well-being, and a shield against depression.

Consider for a moment the elderly preschool teachers Helen Koebert and her two sisters at Messiah Evangelical Lutheran Church in Milwaukee. You won't see their faces on the cover of business magazines. But these energetic and dedicated women, all in their eighties, obtain a deep personal satisfaction from their vital contribution to the life of the faith community that has nurtured them through the difficult periods of their long lives. Knowing they are needed provides them a rich sense of fulfillment that undoubtedly adds to their emotional well-being in healthful ways.

Whatever the undoubtedly complex and multiple causes, however, the apparent health benefits of religion for women in the Strawbridge study were dramatic: When all the factors were statistically weighed, women who were frequent church attenders still had a *34 percent lower hazard of dying* during the study period than women attending services less than once a week. I find the survival-enhancing benefit of this religious involvement quite impressive.

In the years of follow-up, both men and women frequent attenders were much more likely to stop smoking, increase their levels of healthful exercise, enlarge their circles of friends and acquaintances, and increase their membership in nonchurch community groups. These frequent attenders also tended to reduce their drinking during the course of the study more than the less religiously involved people. And during the almost three decades of the study, the regular churchgoers were more likely to stay married to their original spouses than the less frequent attenders.

The researchers did find that healthier lifestyles explained a small but significant proportion of the attendance-survival effect. Certainly, not smoking, cutting back on alcohol, exercising more, and avoiding risky sexual practices—all of which have been connected with religious involvement—may combine to help prevent the onset of some life-threatening diseases.

But the researchers' thorough statistical analysis revealed that all the psychosocial variables (including levels of depression) and healthy lifestyle habits only explained about 30 percent of the attendance-survival connection. So, this left most of this intriguing relationship unexplained. There was something in frequent religious attendance beyond the ready explanations that seemed to protect the most religiously involved.

Another fascinating aspect of this research is that the people studied were in the prime of adult life (age twenty-one to sixty-five), and they came from a part of the country not known for religious activity, as is the Bible Belt.

Finally, the Strawbridge team concluded, the fact that its study found that frequent religious attendance promotes life-enhancing health practices also has "broad public health implications" for the entire country. Religious groups often support health improvement campaigns in their neighborhoods and reach out to "marginal members of their communities." We only need to think of the inspiring experiences of Rick, who was saved from devastating heroin addiction on the blighted streets of North Philadelphia by the Drug Task Force of Deliverance Evangelistic Church, or of Monty Cox, whose conversion and involvement with churches led him from terminal alcoholism to a successful car-repair business that helps restore former substance abusers to productive lives.

The Strawbridge research notes that the prestigious American Public Health Association has set up an initiative to create active partnerships between faith communities nationwide to better coordinate these important efforts.

So, believe me, from a medical researcher's point of view, the evidence of the survival-enhancing benefits of religious involvement that this investigation has uncovered is very significant. All in all, the Alameda County study is one of the best-designed and -conducted pieces of research I've seen in my career.

As in research that we have conducted at Duke, the more religiously involved people in Alameda County reported closer families and friendships, less depression, and healthier lifestyles. Although these elements may combine to help preserve health and extend life, they account for only about one-third of the relationship between religious attendance and survival.

Perhaps the inner peace of deep personal faith combined with the bond of loving concern within a congregation that many religiously active people experience might underpin much of this intriguing suggestion of faith's healing power. The subtle effect of faith on long-term stress reduction, which often leads to better physical health, may be a powerful factor, accounting for some of this otherwise unexplained longevity.

I think it's clear that more research is needed to explore this fascinating connection between religion and prolonged life.

Louise's Story

Louise Hudson is eighty-nine years old. She lives a busy, independent life, driving her own car from her neat home on the shore of Maryland's Chesapeake Bay to a weekly round of fulfilling activities. Her life revolves around church, charity work, regular bus tours with friends, and her responsible position on the county's commission on the aging. Her friends all say that Louise almost radiates a sense of calm and benevolence.

But Louise Hudson's life has not always been so tranquil. She was born in 1909 to a German immigrant mother and an older widower with children who struggled for years to provide a living for his family on a small farm south of Baltimore. Her father died when Louise was only ten, leaving almost no insurance. She went to work as a dime-store clerk, earning seven dollars in pay for a six-day week.

"We were poor," Louise recalls, "but the family stuck together."

Her mother, Anna, had been raised a devout Lutheran in Germany, and instilled her deeply trusting faith in her children.

When the Great Depression swept across the country, Louise found and lost a series of clerking and factory jobs. But she never gave in to pessimism. Her mother had always taught the children to try to learn from adversity and not dwell on problems. Louise married a Baltimore plumber at age twenty-one, but the marriage ended in divorce in 1947. Childless, she found herself a divorced woman in her mid-thirties without a high school diploma and only her own inner strength to sustain her. Once more, her trust in God's benevolence helped preserve her emotional stability.

"I felt somehow that God would not desert me," Louise says of this difficult period.

She earned her high school equivalency diploma, then attended night school to study bookkeeping and later took evening and weekend classes at Loyola University. Louise went to work as a bookkeeper for the State of Maryland in her mid-forties and advanced steadily, taking increasingly responsible positions that had traditionally been filled by men.

Four years later, she married Walter Hudson, a kindly and energetic

man who worked hard as a craftsman and continually sought to improve their life. Louise became a loving mother to Walter's young son,
Jack. It was a pleasant surprise when Walter became an active member
of her church.

After retiring in 1973, Louise looked forward to a time of peaceful
fulfillment with Walter in their secluded home on a branch of the
Chesapeake. But once more, she was confronted by a severe setback.
Walter suffered a devastating stroke that left him almost completely
paralyzed. Louise could have shunted him off to a nursing home, but
chose instead to keep Walter with her at home. At first the stress and
sheer drudgery of caring for a large man confined to either a bed or a
wheelchair almost overwhelmed her. But she fell back on her childhood
religious faith to bolster her strength and courage. Her mother had always taught that God rewarded those who did not give up. And Louise
believed without question that there was a purpose to this painful time.

Despite the strain, she understood that Walter honored her for this
sacrifice. His horizons had narrowed drastically, but Louise was able to
brighten his life. On some warm Indian summer afternoons, she would
wheel his chair to their dock and they'd peacefully watch the graceful,
honking flights of Canada geese returning from the north to winter on
the bay. God had brought Louise and Walter together at a difficult time
in both their lives, she recognized. And God meant her to care for him
as long as she could.

Louise recognized, however, that her own health was not perfect.
Even before she retired, her doctor had detected ominous signs of atherosclerosis, the early stages of coronary artery blockage that often
progress to dangerous levels. An intelligent, well-informed person,
Louise also understood that unmitigated stress and a negative outlook
could exacerbate her heart condition. She intensified her lifelong practice of daily meditative prayer. Her profound faith in God's ultimate
benevolence provided her great emotional comfort, especially during
prayer or scriptural reading.

When Walter died six years later, Louise was deeply saddened, but
satisfied that she had enriched this final, difficult stage of his life. As in
the past, she looked optimistically ahead. Louise, now in her seventies,

devoted much of her time to church activities. Her Woman's Guild at Galilee Lutheran Church helps support a seminary student through regular bake sales and flea markets. She joined a Bible study class led by her pastor, Rev. Chuck Braband, that thoroughly investigated scripture in a manner that Louise found deeply satisfying. It was as if her entire eventful life, with its setbacks and rewards, had prepared her for this spiritual journey.

Louise Hudson's closest friends are members of the Galilee congregation, forming an emotionally nurturing bond of social support that we have seen in research studies of other religious people.

Louise has also become increasingly involved in a Lutheran Mission Association compassion center in Annapolis. This converted storefront building combines a thrift shop with modest apartments for unwed mothers and meeting rooms for drug and alcohol abuse recovery groups. Louise often drives across the wide Bay Bridge to counsel the young women trying to salvage their lives at the compassion center. "I always tell them not to give up," Louise says. She explains to girls still in their teens, struggling to care for a baby and finish high school, that their lives' horizons are much wider than they could ever imagine. "Never forget," she tells the young women, "God will help you in any situation if you reach out."

Now almost ninety, Louise Hudson is aware that her physical strength is beginning to wane. There are many mornings when she finds it difficult to start her busy day. But she always feels better when she completes her morning prayers and launches into her active routine.

"We don't always know what God wants in our lives," she reflects. "But I have to trust that He will help me do what's best."

The Scientific Evidence Builds

Recently, I worked with my colleague David B. Larson, M.D., who also heads the privately funded National Institute for Healthcare Research, to carefully analyze sixty-four research studies on the relationship between religion and mortality, which were published between 1933 and

1995.[2] We wanted to determine if there was consistent evidence that religious faith actually does enhance longevity. As we suspected, the scientific methodology employed in most of the studies, especially the older ones, was too weak to provide the reliable information we needed. Only fifteen of the sixty-four studies actually investigated why and how religion might be related to survival, and most of the fifteen considered only theories about diet and lifestyle.

Despite these shortcomings, however, more than two-thirds of the total studies reported a positive association between religion and survival involving at least one physical illness. Many studies looked at survival advantages among members of traditionally healthy religious groups, such as Seventh-Day Adventists and Mormons, who consistently had lower mortality rates than members of other groups.

An impressive 70 percent of the studies examining church attendance and other measures of religious faith reported longer survival connected to these factors.

In the late 1960s, researcher James House led a team investigating how social relationships and activities were linked with mortality. They studied death from all causes among 2,754 Midwestern men and women between ages thirty-five and sixty-nine for up to twelve years.[3] The team also measured frequency of church attendance, participation in community groups and volunteer associations, and level of visiting with friends and relatives. One significant finding was a connection between church attendance and risk of death among women: 17.3 percent of women who never attended church died, compared with 5.4 percent of the weekly attenders. The general similarity in findings between the House and Strawbridge studies tends to confirm that this type of research has identified a survival-enhancing benefit of religious involvement, at least as seen through the standard measure of frequency of attendance at services.

It's also interesting to note in the House study that the activity "watching TV" was associated with an increased risk of death among the women, indicating again that there is a lot to be said for getting out of the house and becoming active with a church or community group.

A smaller study of elderly poor people in Connecticut also produced interesting results. Researchers from Yale University found that "religiousness" (attendance at worship services, degree of personal faith, and deriving emotional strength from religion) protected the elderly, especially those in worse health. The nonreligious people suffering ill health were almost two and a half times more likely to die than their religious counterparts during the two-year follow-up investigation. Deriving strength from religion was the strongest survival predictor among the three religious variables investigated.[4]

Cancer Protection Among the Conservative Religious

Nationwide, investigators have found provocative evidence that membership in conservative Protestant churches—which exert strong social pressure on members to practice healthy lifestyles—offers significant protection against death from cancer.

University of Florida researcher Jeffrey W. Dwyer and his colleagues studied cancer death rates at the county level, compiled by the National Center for Health Statistics. The team matched information on religious affiliations for these counties. The results were dramatic: Conservative Protestants had lower cancer death rates than liberal Protestants. Counties with higher concentrations of conservative or moderate Protestants had significantly lower mortality from cancer than those with higher concentrations of liberal Protestants. The counties with the highest concentration of Jewish people had the highest cancer death rates, the opposite of counties with high concentrations of Mormons. (The significant impact on cancer mortality rates held for all types of malignancy, not just cancers of the respiratory system strongly associated with smoking, which we might have expected since Mormons do not smoke.)

There are several possible explanations for these findings, including the peer pressure against unhealthy habits that exists within a tightly knit conservative Protestant community, one of the study's main discoveries. The historic trend away from religious observance and synagogue membership among Jews might also account in part for the higher cancer death rates.[5] Research I've helped conduct at Duke has linked strong faith and religious involvement with greater emotional tranquillity and an enhanced sense of well-being. As we will discuss in detail, such inner peace helps maintain a healthy immune system, which may prevent the onset of cancer. It would be interesting to see research similar to studies of secular and observant Jews in Israel conducted among their counterparts in America.

It's only logical that longer life often involves a period of adolescence largely free of serious disease, during which a person practices the healthier habits that many religious people follow as part of their faith. Larson and I concluded that the improved longevity reported in this research could be partly, but not entirely, explained by the healthier diet and less risky lifestyles common to not only Seventh-Day Adventists and Mormons, but also to conservative Protestant congregations.

Some religious groups studied forbid or discourage tobacco and alcohol; most are adamantly opposed to extramarital sex. There also, however, had to be positive prohealth forces at work among the religious people studied. Religious faith may both directly and indirectly (through increased social support) improve health: Faith fosters early disease detection and treatment, anchors healthier lifestyles, and promotes emotional health by mitigating stress and reducing stress-related physical illness.

Please note that I'm not simplistically proposing that religious faith or churchgoing are magic bullets that will prevent the normal decline in physical function we call aging. But ongoing research and a body of published studies at Duke and other institutions do offer convincing evidence that the lives of religiously involved people tend to be both longer and healthier than those of their less religious peers.

And recently, unrelated public health research supported this proposition that the moderate, healthy lifestyle followed by so many people as a matter of faith continues to protect their health and extend longevity as they age. Almost twenty years ago, Stanford University medical professor James F. Fries, M.D., argued that, with improved medical care and better health practices, people would remain healthy and functional until the very end of life, rather than suffer increasing disability as they age.[6] If Fries's theory is valid, it would be good news indeed for millions of people who fear spending their final years disabled in a nursing home.

Religious Faith and Fewer Disabilities

In April 1998, Fries joined a team of researchers who published a follow-up report in the *New England Journal of Medicine* entitled "Aging, Health Risks, and Cumulative Disability."[7] They found that people with "lower health risks," which included not smoking, maintaining a reasonable weight, and getting regular moderate exercise, not only had lower initial levels of disability when they reached older age, but also enjoyed significantly lower "cumulative" disabilities in later life than people who had less healthy lifestyles. Further, the Stanford researchers reported that this healthy longevity was found among both men and women.

This is really excellent news for those Baby Boomers who are working hard to preserve their health, but who still fear that any years added to their lives might be spent in disability and lost independence.

The Stanford report bolstered the findings of a study that Rutgers University researcher Ellen Idler and her Yale University colleague Stanislav Kasl published in the *Journal of Gerontology* in November 1997, which rigorously investigated whether levels of religious involvement influenced changes in physical health, particularly disability, among older people. Their results and conclusions were fascinating.

Idler and Kasl carefully analyzed detailed information collected on 2,812 elderly Catholics, Protestants, and Jews in New Haven, Connecticut, during a twelve-year public survey that began in 1982.[8] They focused on what doctors call "functional ability," the degree to which people could live independently and perform the daily tasks that younger, healthy people take for granted. Selecting among the common impairments of the elderly, the team focused on general disability, stroke with paralysis or related problems, less severe stroke, different levels of diabetes, broken bones (due in part to falls and osteoporosis), amputations, heart disease, and deteriorating mental ability.

Idler and Kasl's central hypothesis was that level of religious involvement, including attendance at church and synagogue, would prove to be connected to better functional ability over the twelve years of the study. They based this view on research, including studies we'd conducted at Duke, which clearly demonstrated that religiously active people have a better overall sense of well-being and meaning in their lives.

The team divided its central hypothesis into several separate lines of inquiry. These included testing whether religious activity would be related to better functioning over time among people whose initial levels of performance were the same. Further, it was thought that disability would cause short-term, but not long-term declines in attendance at religious services. Idler and Kasl also believed that people who had some disability at the start of the study would enjoy the greatest benefits of religious attendance. The effect of attendance at services on functional ability, the researchers thought, might be explained in part by the better health practices and larger circles of friends and more active social networks of frequent service attenders. Finally, the team thought that some of the link between religious attendance and better functional ability would be explained by the higher levels of well-being that have been observed among the frequent attenders.

Idler and Kasl's findings shed a lot of light on the importance of congregational worship among older people—as concerns levels of disability and functional ability—a relationship that many gerontologists and public health specialists ignore.

Level of religious service attendance remained amazingly stable throughout the entire study. At the beginning, 40 percent of the people reported attending services at least once a week; by 1994, even with natural mortality and increasing disability among this elderly group, the weekly or more frequent attendance had only dropped to 38 percent. This insignificant decline in attendance occurred in the face of a much larger overall increase in impaired functioning, which to the researchers suggested that some levels of disability among older people do not prevent them from attending religious services. The joy and bonds of loving friendship that older people have probably experienced throughout their lives at their churches and synagogues obviously outweigh the pain and discomfort of impairment caused by arthritis, heart trouble, partial paralysis, and even amputations.

Thus, people's level of functional disability in 1982 was not related to a decline in their religious attendance in any of the years of the study, once other factors, including original health status, gender, race, and level of social involvement, were considered. During the years of follow-up, disability sometimes presented short-term barriers to attending services among the religiously active, but this could not be detected three years later after the next survey interval. In other words, those people of strong faith who wanted to join their congregations for worship either overcame their disabilities or found ways to accommodate them so that they could again regularly attend services.

To me, a specialist in geriatric psychiatry who has seen a lot of immobilizing discouragement in physically impaired older people, this finding speaks of a powerful motivation among the faithful. And indeed, the researchers found that the extent of one's personal faith was connected to this process. They also found that previous attendance patterns and strong faith were not easily eroded by changes in disability. I am reminded of Marguerite Grounds, who has undergone repeated painful orthopedic surgery which would have kept many people in their eighties bedridden, but who returns to worship at Cheek Height Baptist Church whenever her health permits. Many people I've studied use the term "home church." It is among their congregations that they feel the closest bonds of emotionally warm attachment outside their immediate families. It was this strong tie between fellow worshipers that I believe Idler and Kasl discovered in their research.

The study's other main findings were also compelling. Concerning functional ability, people's frequency of attendance at services in 1982 was a consistent predictor of reduced risk of disability over most of the twelve years of the study. It wasn't until the last few years of the investigation that the general level of disability among those who attended service most frequently in 1982 began to rise to a significant degree. This indicates they enjoyed better functional ability than their less religiously active peers for between six to twelve years of later life.

Researchers did find some connection between the healthier

emotional lives and closer social ties religiously active people often enjoy and their lower levels of disability later in life. They also found that
higher levels of physical activity had an effect on reducing disability
throughout the study, but when analyzed from several statistical perspectives, this did not account for the increased benefits of frequent religious attendance. Nor did leisure and social activities. The authors
concluded: ". . . a significant effect of religiousness remains, even after
social activities have been considered."

Concerning the improved well-being among religiously active people that had been discovered in earlier research, the study found that
the separate element of optimism partially predicted better functioning
later in life. But this too could not explain the complete effect of religious involvement.

Overall, then, one of the strongest predictors of lower disability
throughout the study remained the level of religious attendance in
1982. One of the authors' important conclusions was that "attendance
at religious services plays an important role in predicting the course of
disability that is not accounted for by prior disability or health status"
or other recognized factors, including levels of social activities, better
health practices, or the improved emotional health which research has
shown to be connected to religious involvement.

Idler and Kasl suggest that there are important but subtle factors, including a unique type of personal bonding connected to regular attendance at religious services, which contribute to better health. This
attendance appeared to be a type of "linchpin" that links religious people closely to friends and relatives, to holiday worship and celebrations
that give structure to the year, and to fulfilling social and cultural activities.

Spiritual Joy

But there is also an intense personally satisfying spiritual element in
group worship that goes beyond the ties of loving friendship, the researchers conclude. "Worshipping together with the religious congrega-

tion may offer the disabled elderly person a route through prayer, or receiving the sacraments, or appreciation of the beauty of the place, to a transcendent state in which the body and its frailties don't matter that much."

We only have to think of the transcendental strength Louise Hudson draws from church attendance and receiving communion to recognize the truth of this conclusion.

Idler and Kasl suggest that this transcendental joy, accompanied by the warm support of friends and the enjoyable pastimes religious groups provide, "may be a strong factor influencing the recovery of elderly people with new disabilities."

They also make a relevant point in noting that attendance at religious service is not "a scarce resource," but widely available across the country. And congregational worship is all the more important because religious groups open the door to other health-enhancing, life-promoting resources, particularly for isolated elderly people.

I think it's only logical to assume that the same transcendental peace older people obtain in regular congregational worship plays a role in helping motivate those younger adults and middle-age people who attend religious services to avoid smoking and find time for regular moderate exercise, healthy habits that have proven effective in extending good health throughout a person's elderly years.

As we've seen, emotional health and a sense of well-being promote such beneficial habits. In turn, a healthy mind and body during a person's younger years often extend into a rich and fulfilling later life.

Chapter Eight

✳

Religion May Protect People from Serious Cardiovascular Disease

Afflictions of the heart and blood vessels, commonly called cardiovascular disease, are the leading killer in the developed world. In America alone, over nine hundred thousand people die each year of heart attacks, stroke, and the effects of hypertension (high blood pressure). Cardiovascular disease kills almost twice as many Americans as cancer, annually claiming more lives than the seven next leading causes of death combined.

According to the American Heart Association's most recent statistics, more than fifty-eight million people suffer some form of cardiovascular disease.[1]

Although most people dying of heart disease, stroke, and other cardiovascular disorders are elderly, about 17 percent of these deaths occur before age sixty-five. According to the National Center for Health Statistics, our life expectancy would increase by almost ten years if cardiovascular disease were eliminated.

Coronary heart disease (CHD) involves the intricate web of blood vessels feeding the heart itself and accounts for just over half the total deaths from cardiovascular disease in America. During a heart attack (acute myocardial infarction), vital coronary heart arteries are blocked by clumps of sticky plaque, which our bodies naturally produce from cholesterol, a substance found in all animal cells.

Over 15 percent of the people who die of coronary heart disease— about 74,000 men and women—are under sixty-five years old. This means that medicine simply cannot dismiss CHD as an inevitable consequence of aging, which should cause my Baby Boom generation to seriously consider steps we can take to protect our health as we enter later life.

Over 600,000 Americans annually suffer a first or recurrent stroke. More than 160,000 people die of stroke each year.

When I was a young doctor in training, the prevailing attitude of the medical profession was that cardiovascular disease increased inexorably with age and might be delayed but not eliminated. But as the insightful Stanford University research recently published in the *New England Journal of Medicine* suggests, better health care and health-promoting lifestyle changes can prevent the onset of serious disease until very late in life.

However, even though physicians have an impressive array of medicative and surgical therapies available to treat cardiovascular disease, the actual number of people dying from heart conditions and stroke each year has declined very little since I was a medical student making rounds in the wards of San Francisco General.

Our Risk of Cardiovascular Disease

Hypertension (high blood pressure), which afflicts over fifty million Americans, contributes to cardiovascular disease in several ways. We measure blood pressure in millimeters of mercury: mmHg. An adult blood pressure of 120/80 mmHg (systolic/diastolic) is the ideal. Systolic, the higher number, is recorded when the heart contracts to pump; the diastolic reading, the lower number, is measured when the heart briefly relaxes between beats.

Hypertension—especially high diastolic pressure—is associated with a greater risk of heart attack, due in part to the damage high blood pressure causes to the walls of the coronary arteries that feed our vital heart muscle. One type of damage is a "nidus," a small tear or lesion where plaque made up of cholesterol products and components of our blood can build up to form a blockage. High blood pressure is also connected to heart failure, which occurs when the heart muscle strains to pump blood against increased vascular resistance. This can lead to an enlarged, weakened heart. The important fact to bear in mind about high diastolic blood pressure is that this is the pressure that the heart and the entire vascular system must endure twenty-four hours a day—unlike systolic blood pressure, which occurs only intermittently with each heartbeat.

High blood pressure is also a leading cause of stroke. When combined with a history of heart disease and smoking, high blood pressure is much more likely to trigger stroke in relatively younger people (under age sixty-five) than when found as an independent risk factor.

The American Heart Association has recently begun calling stroke "brain attack," both to alert people to its deadly potential and to describe its physical causes. Most strokes, like heart attacks, are caused by a blockage of a critical artery. Plaque and blood clots can either form in a brain artery or drift there from elsewhere in the body to lodge at a narrow bend or juncture, depriving the vulnerable brain tissue "downstream" of oxygenated blood. A smaller proportion of strokes are hemorrhagic, caused by a burst vessel wall or the failure of a pouchlike aneurysm. The results of all types of stroke are similar: Brain tissue deprived of life-giving blood begins to die within minutes and paralysis of varying extent and severity occurs, depending on the side of the brain infarcted (blocked).

We have about four million surviving stroke victims, the majority with some type of impairment ranging from partial to complete paralysis and often including blindness, inability to speak, and, devastated cognitive power up to complete dementia.

People have high blood pressure for a variety of reasons, including their diet, level of physical activity, weight and body mass, and the way they normally cope with stress. Blood pressure also tends to gradually increase with age in later life. Besides contributing to cardiovascular disease, high blood pressure can affect our other organs, especially the kidneys.

Our bodies' manner of processing the fat we eat, as measured in tests for serum lipids, also affects our relative risk of developing cardiovascular disease. Most of us know that a "high" cholesterol level (over 200 mg/dl) is unhealthy, but rely on doctors to explain the relationship between the "bad" LDL cholesterol to the "good" HDL on our blood tests. In general, a diet high in saturated animal fat and hydrogenated polyunsaturated vegetable fat (think of stick margarine) and low in whole grains, fruits, and vegetables can increase our serum lipids to dangerous levels and make us more vulnerable to cardiovascular disease.

Obesity, usually resulting from the combination of a high-calorie, high-fat diet and too little physical activity, is a prominent cardiovascular disease risk factor.

We've gotten used to thinking of cigarette smoking as the major preventable cause of lung cancer, which it is. But many of us don't realize that smoking is also a leading contributor to cardiovascular disease. Two of every five smoking-related deaths is from heart or vascular disease or stroke.

Today, however, medical science has proven that our risk of suffering cardiovascular disease can often be reduced through changes in lifestyle that include not smoking, eating a healthy diet, cutting back on alcohol, watching our weight, and getting regular exercise.

And now there is also indisputable scientific evidence that unrelieved stress and depression can seriously damage our cardiovascular health. So, by reducing the impact of stress and avoiding the onset of major depression, we can also help preserve our cardiovascular health.

Stress and Your Heart

We all confront some degree of stress in our daily lives. But serious negative events—physical illness, conflicts at work and among family members—can produce chronic stress over months and years. How we deal with this type of stress can affect our risk of developing cardiovascular disease.

Most of us learned in high school about the fight-or-flight response, which is literally programmed into all complex animal species, including homo sapiens. It's an evolutionary survival adaptation that gave our forebears the strength and speed needed to spear a mammoth or, equally important, to flee from predators such as saber-toothed tigers. Now, in the age of freeways and Monday morning department meetings, we've retained this primitive survival mechanism.

Think of the last time you were behind the wheel of a car on a crowded highway and some aggressive driver cut you off, jamming in so fast and close that you had to hit the brakes to avoid a collision. Can you recall that instant flood of sensation that tingled painfully hot and cold through your throat and face? Can you still feel your hands clenching desperately, the tension in your back and legs, the alarming thud of your heart, the gasp as your lungs filled?

What we can't see, of course, are the "stress hormones" flooding our bodies. These hormones—cortisol, epinephrine, and norepinephrine—produced by the adrenal glands near the kidneys, are potent chemical messengers. When we're stimulated by actual physical danger, perceived aggression in others, or anticipation of an unpleasant confrontation, stress hormones are released and our bodies react involuntarily.

In extreme cases, our cardiovascular and respiratory systems jump into emergency passing gear. When stress hormones stimulate the autonomic nervous system, our heart rate shoots up, our lungs expand, and our breathing becomes rapid. Our muscles tense and blood vessels contract—even as the actual flow of blood increases—suddenly raising blood pressure. Our blood platelets become more sticky and clump together to minimize bleeding in case of injury.

Few people confront extreme physical danger in today's world, but stressful situations assail us in normal life. Under the threat of downsizing, productivity has become increasingly important in factory and office. Many people suffer the gnawing stress of too much work and too little time to complete it. Trying to balance the demands of work and family life can lead to the "burnout" so many working mothers experience.

We all recognize the discomfort of sudden stressful encounters, especially if we're powerless to either fight or flee—when the boss berates us, or when we are harassed by aggressive drivers. However, prolonged, unmitigated stress can trigger depression, and this can lead to cardiovascular disease and even a fatal heart attack.

In some people suffering chronic emotional tension, vascular plaque builds up at vulnerable sites in coronary arteries that have been repeatedly constricted by the effect of stress hormones. The heart muscle is deprived of oxygen-rich blood and chest pain (angina) ensues. Sometimes the pulsing heart muscle slips into chaotic arrhythmia and death occurs. Such sudden cardiac death is more common than most of us realize. Over 350,000 of our fellow Americans suffer this fate annually.

Religious Faith and Stress Management

But is cardiovascular disease caused by chronic stress and depression an inevitable by-product of our hectic world? Is there any practical way we can defuse the bioevolutionary time bomb of the fight-or-flight response?

Yes, possibly so. Research has found that religious faith and practices such as prayer, scriptural reading, and attendance at worship service may help diminish the impact of emotional stress in daily life and mitigate the more severe stress of illness. As we've seen, people with religious faith are also protected from depression.

Louise Hudson's potentially serious atherosclerosis, detected in middle age, never progressed to serious proportions. Her cardiovascular health is in fact excellent for a woman almost ninety. This is especially impressive because she endured prolonged stress during her husband's disability, then suffered potentially depressing bereavement on his death. Louise has also grieved the recent deaths of her stepson Jack and his wife. Throughout her life, religious faith has mitigated the stress of uncertainty and major setbacks. But can we say with certainty that faith has preserved her cardiovascular health? Once more, Louise's story is a strong anecdotal account of faith's healing power. But for scientific evidence, we must turn to the findings of systematic research.

Researchers theorize that the inner peace found in religion may lower the production of stress hormones, which in turn calms the autonomic nervous system, decreasing heart rate, vascular tension, and dangerous platelet clotting. Faith and religious practice may also help prevent high blood pressure and thus reduce stroke and heart disease. There is evidence, too, that the stress relief inherent in religion lowers the desire to seek emotional comfort through tobacco and alcohol.

LaVerne's Story

In 1992, LaVerne Emery, then seventy-five, was almost ready to surrender to heart disease. In the previous two years, the Milwaukee widow, who had always been outgoing and energetic, had seen her life become increasingly constrained by the unmistakable symptoms of progressive atherosclerotic coronary artery blockage. Walking along the bike path on the bluff above Lake Michigan, which had once been her favorite exercise, had become frightening as her chest would be seized by the cold grip of angina and she'd find herself panting.

For years LaVerne had been active in her church, Ascension Lutheran—a member of the Altar Guild, a hospital visitor who prayed and administered Communion to sick members of the congregation, and a cheerful greeter at Sunday services. Retired for over ten years and living in a comfortable lakeside condominium, LaVerne had spent much of her free time driving older, less fit church friends to services and shopping areas.

But, inexorably, her involvement with church became increasingly constrained as the symptoms of heart disease worsened. LaVerne had always trusted in God to see her through physical illness and provide emotional strength during stressful periods. Her trusting faith, however, simply did not seem adequate to overcome this latest, and most severe, health crisis.

"I'm recommending an angioplasty," her doctor told her after studying the results of a heart catheterization performed in February 1992 which revealed extensive blockage in one of her main coronary arteries.

LaVerne took the news quietly, but felt an inner sense of dread. She well understood the gravity of her condition, having lost her husband to a sudden, premature heart attack years earlier. In fact, the nitroglycerin tablets her doctor had prescribed to ease the pain of angina had become as much an emotional as a physical comfort, and LaVerne felt dread if she ever misplaced the small enamel pillbox containing the medication.

As with previous hospitalizations, LaVerne prepared herself spiritually before she underwent the balloon angioplasty meant to open the blocked heart artery. And for several weeks the procedure seemed to have been successful. Then, only two months later, she felt a stabbing constriction in her chest as she carried a basket of wash to the laundry room of her building. *Oh no*, she thought, half in prayer, half in anguish, *don't let it happen again*.

But, in fact, LaVerne had to endure two more balloon angioplasties on the blocked artery over the coming months (three is the maximum number of these procedures generally recommended on a single artery). Before each of these hospital stays, LaVerne prayed, read scripture, and made a resolution to place all of her trust in God to protect her.

After her third angioplasty in less than a year, she had to rely heavily on that faith to maintain a semblance of her innate optimism. Undergoing cardiac rehabilitation, she was urged by her physical therapist to take up regular, moderate exercise, a key component in preventing further blockage to the coronary arteries.

"That won't be easy," she told the young woman. LaVerne's right knee was swollen and painful from chronic arthritis.

"Well," the therapist suggested, "water walking is a good alternative, and lap swimming is even better."

There was a pool at LaVerne's building, but she had not used it much. She had an unreasonable fear of water, especially when she'd find herself out of her depth with her face beneath the surface. On the few occasions she'd actually tried swimming, either in a pool or at the church's camp on a quiet inland lake, she had come close to outright panic.

So, with arthritis preventing conventional exercise and her water phobia ruling out use of the pool, LaVerne's normal optimistic outlook narrowed. She began losing interest in church and spent more time alone in her condominium. Some days she didn't even bother to dress or cook a regular meal.

Then, one spring afternoon in 1993 as she parked her car in her building's basement garage after a shopping trip, LaVerne had a sudden insight. God had not withdrawn His interest in her life, or His protection. But she herself had to make an effort to make use of that grace.

"It's only five floors," she told herself as she bypassed the elevator and began slowly, painfully climbing the stairs. That first day she paused at every landing, shifting her small sack of groceries from hand to hand and massaging her arthritic knee. But within a week she could climb an entire one-story flight of stairs without becoming severely winded.

As summer approached, she made another major decision. Her fear of water, she realized, was irrational. On a visit to her daughter on the East Coast, LaVerne enrolled in swimming lessons at a local community college. The first few sessions were frightening, especially when the teacher quietly insisted LaVerne learn to submerge her entire face, hold her breath, and become comfortable in a floating position. But LaVerne overcame her panic and stuck with the lessons.

Seven years after her last angioplasty, LaVerne Emery, now eighty-two, lives with her daughter and son-in-law and has become active in several local churches in her new community. She also swims slow, steady laps in an Olympic-size pool at the college for a full forty-five minutes, three days a week, throughout the year. The regular exercise has not only helped keep her heart healthy, but has also brought dramatic improvement to her arthritic knee.

At her last medical checkup, LaVerne's physician studied the laboratory test printouts and EKG graph. "You're much healthier than most people your age," the doctor said with a smile.

"I didn't do it on my own," LaVerne replied, returning the smile.

Science, Religion, and Your Heart

Investigations I took part in at Duke University and research at other institutions has shown that religious people may be protected from some cardiovascular diseases.

As mentioned, a large, multiyear investigation recently completed by Duke University researchers demonstrates that people for whom religion is important, who attend church, and who regularly pray or read scripture, have lower blood pressure than their less religiously active counterparts.

I became interested in the relationship between religious faith and blood pressure in the 1980s when I joined Dr. David Larson and other colleagues to investigate whether there was any beneficial effect on the blood pressure among frequent churchgoers and on those who found religion important in their lives. We studied 407 men in a rural Georgia county who had earlier been found free of cardiovascular disease or hypertension.

We examined several aspects of their religious lives, including frequency of church attendance, ranging from "daily" to "never." From these we sorted out "high attenders" (those attending at least weekly) and "low attenders." Then we looked at the importance of religion in these men's lives, dividing them into two groups: "high importance" and "low importance."

The original blood pressure readings had been taken three times over a period of an hour by trained research staff, so we were confident they were accurate.

The results were intriguing: Diastolic blood pressures of men with high church attendance and who found religion important in their lives were significantly lower than those of the men in the group that found religion of low importance and who attended church less frequently.

These differences in blood pressure remained after we adjusted for age, body-mass index (a comparison of weight and height) socioeconomic status, and smoking. To our surprise, we found that, especially among smokers, the more religious (high importance) had lower average blood pressure than their less religious peers. In the group of men aged fifty-five and older, the mean difference in the religious men's diastolic blood pressure was clinically significant (6 mmHg lower). Remember, diastolic blood pressure reflects the underlying tension in the vascular system and is an important risk factor in both heart disease and stroke.

Most studies before this one had used church attendance as the key factor in measuring a person's religious faith. We chose to also look at personal perception of religion's importance. We concluded that both religious attitudes and involvement (as reflected in church attendance) may reduce average blood pressure in men.[2]

These findings were interesting, but before reaching any general conclusions about the beneficial effect of religion on blood pressure, I wanted to investigate a larger group of both men and women, over a longer period.

Blood Pressure and Religious Activity

So I helped form a team at Duke University that examined the relationship between religious activities and blood pressure in almost four thousand men and women age sixty-five and older who'd participated in a study sponsored by the National Institutes of Health. We chose this age group because the negative impact of cardiovascular disease becomes increasingly severe in later life.

We recognized from other research at Duke that there was a link between religious involvement and better emotional health, including improved coping with stressful events, especially among older adults. Given the connection between stress and blood pressure, we thought that a greater level of religious activity, which reduces stress and enhances coping, might be associated with lower blood pressure in this large, diverse group.

Through random selection, we chose 3,963 people who had begun the health survey in 1986. The participants underwent in-person interviews conducted by trained research assistants, who gathered information on age, race, schooling, religious activity and denomination, overall physical health, history of cigarette smoking, body-mass index, and blood pressure.[3]

The interviewers asked how often the people attended religious meetings and services, and how frequently they prayed or studied the Bible.

We looked at blood pressure in two ways. First, interviewers asked people if their doctors had ever told them they had high blood pressure. Those answering yes were asked if they were currently taking blood pressure medication. Then the people's systolic and diastolic blood pressures were carefully measured twice, with the initial reading discarded because people feel stressed when a blood pressure cuff is first slipped over their arm.

These interviews and examinations continued in three "waves" over the next six years and included as many of the original group's survivors as remained available.

We were testing several theories about the relationship between religion and blood pressure. Once more, the results were interesting, but slightly different from what we had originally assumed they would be.

First, we thought blood pressures in general would be lower among the more religiously active. This hypothesis was supported for some religious activities, but not others. The number of people whose doctors told them they had high blood pressure was lower among the frequent religious service attenders than among their counterparts who attended infrequently. This held true through all three waves of the study, but after other factors were considered, the differences became insignificant at Waves I and II. At Wave III (1992–94), however, people who attended religious service at least once a week were 8 percent less likely to have been told they had high blood pressure.

When we compared *actual* blood pressure measurements with religious attendance, we found that both systolic and diastolic pressures were significantly lower among frequent attenders than among people who went to religious service less often. Measured blood pressures were also lower for people who regularly prayed or studied the Bible compared with those who were less involved in such activities. This was particularly true for diastolic blood pressure taken at Waves I and III.

In some groups, frequency of religious attendance at one wave predicted lower diastolic blood pressure at later waves, even after taking into consideration all the other social and health factors and baseline blood pressure.

When we examined age and religious attendance, we found that it was among the *younger* elderly (under age seventy-five) that frequent religious service attendance at Wave II was associated with significantly lower blood pressures at Wave III, three years later.

Among black people, both high religious attendance and high levels of private prayer and Bible study at Wave II predicted significantly lower blood pressures three years later at Wave III, after taking account of other factors and baseline blood pressures.

So, high religious activity at one point in time could predict lower blood pressures several years later among the younger elderly and blacks in our study.

We also carefully analyzed our findings to make sure they weren't skewed simply because religious people took their high blood pressure medication more diligently than others.

The more religiously active people *consistently* had 1–4 mmHg lower average blood pressure than infrequent religious service attenders. While this difference is seemingly small, we found that it is clinically significant since cardiovascular risk increases with even small rises in blood pressure. And the *majority* of deaths from high blood pressure occur at levels below the current recommended treatment "thresholds."

Another hypothesis was that diastolic blood pressures would be lowest among people who *both* frequently attended religious services and regularly prayed or studied the Bible. We measured all combinations of these activities and put them through a rigorous statistical test to make sure of our results. The hypothesis was supported in every combination.

After dividing all the subjects into groups with diastolic pressure of 90 mmHg or higher (clinically, *diastolic hypertension*) and diastolic pressures of less than 90 mmHg, we applied standard statistical methods to search for the effects of religious attendance and private prayer and Bible study on the likelihood of diastolic hypertension.

Exciting Results

Taking into consideration all the separate variables, we found that the men and women who *both* attended religious service and prayed or studied the Bible frequently were *40 percent less likely to have diastolic hypertension* than those who attended services and prayed or read the Bible infrequently. The likelihood of this finding occurring simply by "chance" alone was less than 1 in 10,000, which makes the association between religious activity and lower diastolic blood pressure statistically significant and clinically important.

As in any serious scientific study, we wanted to take an honest look at factors that might possibly have skewed our results. We considered the fact that our subjects came from the Bible Belt South, meaning that they were probably more religiously inclined than people from other regions. But research conducted by leading institutions like the Gallup organization has proven that older Americans around the country are generally quite religious, similar to the people in our study.

After taking into consideration all the important factors, the major finding of our study remained: There was substantial *decrease in the likelihood of diastolic hypertension* among the most religiously involved.

Strong evidence suggests that reduction of the American population's mean blood pressure by as little as 2–4 mmHg could reduce cardiovascular disease by 10 to 20 percent. Such a reduction would have a major impact on public health in this country. Remember, the American Heart Association estimates that fifty-eight million Americans have some type of cardiovascular disease, which claims the lives of almost a million people a year. Dramatic reduction in diastolic blood pressure of up to 40 percent could save even more lives. If religious involvement can reduce the blood pressure toll, as our study suggests, we will have found important new evidence of the healing power of faith.

       *

Protection from Heart Attacks

To many people, cardiovascular disease among the elderly is associated with heart attacks. And for good reason. Almost 85 percent of the people who die of coronary heart disease are age sixty-five or older. But the great majority of those under sixty-five who die of myocardial infarction succumb to their first heart attack.

 Can religious faith and involvement protect us from fatal heart disease as well as high blood pressure?

Bernice Graham's Faith and Survival

I recently became acquainted with Bernice Freeman Graham, an emotionally healthy and spiritually strong woman of seventy-five. Bernice's story complements LaVerne Emery's spiritual journey, but reveals an even stronger link between faith and survival.

 Like LaVerne, Bernice Freeman Graham was born into a struggling rural family. The Freemans farmed a few acres of corn and cotton in the North Carolina Piedmont. Bernice was one of nine children, and worked hard in the fields and kitchen garden from early childhood. Her parents were devout members of the local Freewill Baptist Church, which she proudly recalls her "daddy helped build, walls and roof."

 Of Native American ancestry, Bernice grew up amid intolerance and in abject poverty. But her family's bond of love and spirituality was rich and warm. Bernice helped work the land until the 1950s, when she took a job as an upholsterer in a small family-owned furniture shop. These were nonunion days, and piecework was exhausting drudgery that extracted a physical toll.

 "Nobody spends so many years hunched over, tugging and fixing upholstery, without it leaving them bent and sore the rest of their life," she said recently. She made this assessment without rancor or bitterness, however, a sign of her basic optimism.

 She became an especially devout Christian in the 1960s and formed

*

a gospel-song duet with her mother, Emma Lee. Bernice married late in life, at age forty-five, and was widowed early, at only fifty, in 1974. She became the sole support of her small daughter, Cledell. When Bernice moved to work in Lumberton, North Carolina, she missed the close friendships of her home church, which was more like an extended family than a traditional congregation. But she later found great comfort in a new church, Faith of Calvary. Bernice loved both to sing hymns and to lose herself in spiritual joy during long gospel concerts. She was proud when she'd be joined by Cledell, a bright-faced little girl among the swaying women behind the altar.

The years of poverty and struggle had indeed left their mark, however, and Bernice developed serious cardiovascular disease in her fifties. She had two relatively minor heart attacks in 1986, and a brief stroke a year later. Then, on a hot July afternoon in 1995, Bernice suffered a series of severe angina attacks while she was driving her oldest grandchild, Emily Marie, to a swimming class. Somehow she managed to drive home safely before blacking out briefly.

When she underwent catheterization at the local hospital, the cardiologist bent over the table, his eyes anxious above his surgical mask. "Mrs. Graham," he said gently, "we have to get you up to Duke for surgery."

He pointed toward the video monitor and explained that the chalky web on the screen represented her main coronary arteries, which were almost completely blocked by atherosclerosis.

Bernice glanced at the image, then looked back at the concerned young man and smiled. "I'm in the Lord's hands," she said confidently. "I always have been."

The next day as she was wheeled into the operating room for a quadruple bypass, Bernice found herself comforting the nurses and surgeons. "The Lord *will* take care of me," she assured the ring of faces hovering above the gurney.

In fact, Bernice made a remarkably fast recovery, and was released from the hospital five days after this major cardiac surgery. Recuperating at home, she suffered none of the anxiety that afflicts so many postoperative heart patients. She had absolute faith that the outcome of her illness was in God's hands. That faith stood up to a sudden setback the next week when she again blacked out from angina. Tests revealed that two of the bypasses had become blocked with atherosclerotic plaque. Bernice again assured her doctors, "The good Lord will take care of me."

Her physical condition has actually not improved dramatically since her surgery. In May 1997, she collapsed once more from angina, which was traced to slowly progressing arterial blockage. Despite these setbacks, however, Bernice remains calm and cheerfully optimistic. She manages to attend church several times a week, and still sings in the choir. Like Louise Hudson, Bernice begins each day with intense personal prayer, then spends a few minutes reading the Bible. Whenever she feels physically weak, she sits and slowly works her way through a few psalms from the Book of David. "This gives me strength," she says.

The high point of Bernice's week is the long Sunday service, and the chance to join the congregation in song worship. Recently, Bernice was walking slowly but steadily from the church with the congregation surrounding her when her youngest granddaughter, Engliss, a bright and energetic girl of six, took her hand. "Grandma," the child said, "you know I pray for you every night."

Bernice bent and kissed Engliss, filled with the warm certainty that the loving God of her own childhood would never fail to answer those prayers.

Faith and Heart Disease: The Scientific Evidence

Research has shown that people such as Bernice who have strong religious faith and active involvement in faith communities are less likely to die from coronary artery disease, have fewer heart attacks, and live longer after open-heart surgery than their less religious peers.

One of the most compelling of these recent studies on the heart was conducted by Israeli and American investigators led by Uri Goldbourt, Ph.D., and published in the prestigious journal *Cardiology* in 1993. The

team studied death from coronary heart disease among 10,059 male Israeli civil servants and municipal employees over twenty-three years.
Because so many subjects were studied over such a long period, the scientific validity of the findings is increased.

The researchers were trying to identify possible long-term factors
that might predict fatal heart disease, or conversely, habits and
lifestyles that could protect men from this threat. To minimize the effect of genetic predisposition toward either good or bad cardiovascular
health, the researchers chose Jewish men born in different parts of Europe, the Middle East, and North Africa as well as native-born sabras
from Palestine. All the participants were aged forty or over and underwent a thorough medical examination in 1963. They were also interviewed about their religious education and upbringing and any
experience they might have had during the Holocaust.

The men answered several questions about their religion. They
noted whether they were educated in religious or secular schools or
both, stated how often they went to synagogue, and defined their level
of religious faith. With this information, the researchers developed an
"orthodoxy" scale that ranged from secular to orthodox.

During the twenty-three years of the study (1963–86), 1,098 of the
men died from coronary heart disease. Those born in the Middle East
outside of Palestine and those from North African countries had the
lowest rates of heart disease death, the men from eastern and southeast-
ern Europe the highest.

As expected, several physical health factors seemed to predict death
from heart disease. These included low blood levels of what we often
call "good" (HDL) cholesterol. In general, higher average blood pressure (especially when combined with lower levels of HDL) increased
the risk of heart disease. Cigarette smoking was also a major risk factor.

After taking into consideration all of the separate health and social
factors, the researchers found a definite connection between the participants' "degree of religious orthodoxy" and their coronary heart disease
(CHD) death rates. "The highly orthodox religious groups of the
study experienced significantly reduced CHD death rates" when
compared with the other participants, the researchers noted. The

protective quality of religious faith also held for other causes of death among the men studied. (This finding was similar to the results of the research on the religious and secular kibbutzim which we looked at earlier.)

Uri Goldbourt's research team found that the apparent protective value of religious orthodoxy held through the different national-origin groups of the men studied. This is significant, because many of the Middle Eastern and North African Jews had a genetic background somewhat different from that of the predominantly Ashkenazi men born in Europe.

The researchers found that the "most orthodox" men in the study retained a reduced long-term CHD death risk compared with that of the less religious, secular, and "nonbelievers" when all the important health factors—including average systolic blood pressure, total cholesterol, diabetes, and even cigarette smoking—were statistically taken into account.

Very exciting and significant is the fact that the most religious men had a *20 percent lower risk of death from CHD* over the years of the study compared with the other groups.

For example, in the recent study on the relationship between religious activity and cigarette smoking that our Duke team conducted, we found that smokers aged sixty-five and older were 54 percent more likely to die during the study period than nonsmokers.[4] If active religious involvement can reduce heart disease death risk by a minimum of 20 percent among adults, this has major public health implications.

The Israeli researchers also noted that mortality from all natural causes was "significantly reduced in the 'most orthodox' individuals."

The men studied had "lived in years of political and social turmoil," an understatement when you consider the Holocaust and all the wars since Israeli independence. The period of the study was obviously a time of great stress. But the most orthodox men were better protected from fatal heart disease during this period than their less observant peers.

This protective aspect of the orthodox life probably stems from the stress reduction inherent in deep faith and membership in a devout community. Orthodox Jews pray several times a day. They participate in emotionally moving worship service at least twice each Sabbath and spend the remainder of that day with their families. The orthodox year is punctuated by religious holidays, some, such as Yom Kippur, profoundly spiritual. The orthodox draw great personal comfort from scripture, especially the Psalms. Many orthodox Jewish men feel an intense personal connection to an all-powerful God who intervenes directly in their lives. This transcendental connection, regularly reinforced throughout the liturgical year, helps keep the stress of daily life in perspective.

There is solid scientific evidence that other forms of religious faith may offer similar protection.

Social Support and Heart Surgery

One of the more interesting research studies of this phenomenon in America was led by Dr. Thomas Oxman of the Dartmouth Medical School and published in the journal *Psychosomatic Medicine* in 1995.[5] Oxman and his colleagues were interested in the relationship between social support and religion on the one hand and death among older patients following open-heart surgery on the other. The researchers had noted that there was substantial scientific evidence on the physical health factors influencing patients' survival after heart surgery and that there was a growing body of research on social factors such as marital status, emotional support from family and friends, and personality.

Oxman's team found that emotional support from social groups such as friends from work or clubs was likely to decrease as a person aged. But involvement in religion often takes the place of this emotional support among the elderly.

And because studies of survival of elderly cardiac surgery patients had largely overlooked the influence of social support and religion on postsurgical survival, the researchers decided to focus on this intriguing area.

Using a rigorous scientific approach, the researchers selected 232 patients age fifty-five and older who were undergoing elective heart surgery for artery bypass grafts, aortic valve replacement, or both. The patients were contacted before surgery and interviewed by an experienced psychiatrist to assess their emotional health, the extent of their social support networks, and their religious beliefs and practices. The patients were also tested for depressive symptoms. During this presurgical period, the patients underwent a full battery of physical health examinations, with a thorough investigation of their cardiac condition.

The interviewers asked five specific questions on the scope of the patients' religious involvement, concerning their denomination, the patterns of their attendance at religious functions, their social contacts within their faith community, the strength and comfort they receive from their religious faith, and finally, their overall sense of religiousness.

Within six months of surgery, twenty-one of the original patients had died—twenty from cardiovascular disease, one from lung cancer. The researchers carefully analyzed the social support and religion factors of both the patients who had died and those who had survived.

Some highly provocative findings resulted. After adjusting for biomedical risk factors, the elderly patients who were both socially active and found strength and comfort in their religious faith were *fourteen times less likely to die* during the six months following surgery than their counterparts who lacked social support and the emotional bolstering of religious faith. The emotional sustenance patients found in religion was independently protective. "Among the religion variables," the researchers noted, "those without any strength and comfort from religion had almost three times the risk of death as those with at least some strength and comfort."

Equally intriguing, the investigators found that of the thirty-seven patients in the original group who'd said they were "deeply" religious, none died during the six-month follow-up period. And among the hundred patients who reported attending religious service "at least every few months," only five (5 percent) died, giving them about one-half the death rate of those who reported "never or rarely" attending services. The study also found that patients without religious strength and comfort also had fewer close emotional social connections and were less likely to be married. But, despite those related social support factors, the researchers concluded that absence of strength and comfort was the only religion variable "uniquely related to mortality."

Discussing hypotheses to explain the possible protective qualities of religious faith, the team noted that strong traditional belief and group guidance toward a healthy lifestyle among a congregation might result in less smoking and drinking, a benefit to cardiac health. "However, in this study," the researchers stated, "there were no differences in smoking status [smoker versus nonsmoker] between those with absence of strength and comfort from religion and those with the presence of strength and comfort from religion." This suggests that there was some element in deep religious faith beyond a healthier lifestyle that explained the protective effects among the more devoutly religious patients.

The findings also suggested there was a protective cardiac health benefit in receiving "at least a little strength and comfort" from religious faith.

Reinforcing the conclusions of this study is another intriguing investigation from Israel, this one examining the relationship between religious orthodoxy and heart attack (myocardial infarction) incidence among secular and orthodox Jewish people in Jerusalem suffering their first heart attack. This group was compared with a larger group that was free of heart disease. Secular people had a significantly higher risk of myocardial infarction than did orthodox subjects. *Among secular men, the heart attack risk was three to seven times greater; in the women studied, the risk ranged from two to twenty-three times greater.*[6] In a related later study of young Jewish people ages seventeen and eighteen, Yechiel Friedlander's team found that blood levels of total cholesterol, triglycerides, and "bad" (LDL) cholesterol were higher among youth from secular families than in youth from orthodox families. Analysis showed that intensity of religious observance played a role in the lower cholesterol among the orthodox young people.[7]

Based on this accumulation of research findings, it appears that religious faith and practice may not only lower the risk of serious heart disease, but also help promote survival when a person already has a life-threatening heart condition.

Only a few years ago, when I'd discuss the enduring faith of patients like Bernice Graham with my medical colleagues, some of them would indulge me with a noncommittal smile and politely change the subject. After all, faith was a supernatural matter, and the progression or remission of cardiovascular disease was a scientific issue. Recently, however, my surgeon, cardiologist, and internist friends are beginning to pay more attention to the relationship between emotional health supported by faith and cardiovascular disease among their patients. This shift in attitude is based in part on new evidence that there is a strong link between depression and coronary heart disease.

Depression and Coronary Heart Disease

In 1993, Canadian researcher Nancy Frasure-Smith, Ph.D., and her colleagues published a major study about depression, heart attack, and survival in the *Journal of the American Medical Association*.[8] They wanted to determine if medically diagnosed depression in patients hospitalized following a heart attack would influence their death from heart disease—independent of other factors—during the first six months after leaving the hospital. They interviewed 222 heart attack patients at the Montreal Heart Institute, carefully screening them for symptoms of major depression. Thirty-five were diagnosed with major depressive illness.

Within six months of discharge from the Heart Institute, a total of twelve of the original patients had died of cardiac causes. Significantly, the dead included six of the depressed people, half the mortalities, even though only 16 percent of the original group of 222 had been diagnosed with depression.

The Canadian researchers carefully compared all the other risk factors, including social and marital status, smoking history, severity of cardiac illness, and damage to the heart. They found that *major depression in these heart attack patients was an independent risk factor for higher mortality.* The depressed patients "were at significantly greater risk of dying over the subsequent six months than patients who were not depressed," the investigators commented, adding that their study was the first to demonstrate "an independent impact of major depression" on the prognosis of heart attack victims.

The researchers concluded that depressed people have often lost interest in life and might be less likely to follow medical guidance and adopt a healthier lifestyle.

Comparing these people with Louise Hudson and Bernice Graham, whose positive attitudes are based in large measure on their religious faith, we can begin to make a connection between the protection from depression religion provides and cardiovascular health.

Indeed, the Canadian team cited current research suggesting two mind-body mechanisms that help explain the link between depression and death after heart attack. As we described earlier, severe stress and depression disturb the autonomic nervous system in ways similar to the fight-or-flight response. Also, depression can make blood platelets stickier and more likely to clump. This aspect of depression appears connected to fluctuations in the brain chemical serotonin, the activity of which becomes increasingly disrupted as depression increases.

Although the Canadian study was limited in size, the researchers' scientific methods were rigorous. But can we apply their conclusions more widely?

Depression and Increased Risk

In January 1998, Alexander H. Glassman, M.D., a world-renowned expert in the effects of drug treatments on depression among heart disease patients, and his colleague at Columbia University, Peter A. Shapiro, M.D., published an important report on depression and coronary heart disease in the *American Journal of Psychiatry.*[9] Carefully analyzing ten recent research studies, Glassman and Shapiro noted that nine of them found increased mortality from cardiovascular disease among depressed patients. Just in the past two years, the researchers found, five of six community health surveys following people initially free of heart ailments have noted an increased risk of coronary heart disease among those with depression.

Glassman and Shapiro noted that the increased risk of cardiovascular disease in depressed people was not due to smoking or other known risk factors such as weight, level of physical activity, blood pressure, gender, or cholesterol levels. "We found that the apparently healthy individuals who had elevated depression ratings were more likely to develop and die of ischemic [blocked artery] heart disease," the researchers emphasized. They cited recent research in Baltimore that found "a diagnosis of major depression increased the risk of myocardial infarction more than fourfold after control for medical risk factors and other psychiatric diagnoses."

Chronic changes in the tone of the autonomic nervous system, so often seen in serious depression, appeared to be associated with increased heart attack risk. But Glassman and Shapiro also highlighted ongoing research showing the impact of depression on blood platelets and the increased risk of coronary artery blockage by the resulting plaque deposits. Research on people who suffered sudden cardiac death suggested that almost a quarter of them were suffering "substantial emotional distress" just before they died.

Glassman and Shapiro's careful analysis also undercut the established view that a "type A" personality is especially prone to heart disease. Such a person, who used to be called "a heart attack waiting to happen," is impatient, competitive, and often reacts with irritation under stress. But the researchers found that thorough investigations conducted over years actually showed that depression, not a type A personality, was the more accurate predictor of cardiovascular disease risk.

"Our review of the evidence," the Columbia researchers concluded, "suggests that depression is a major contributor to heart disease and that the two conditions in later life may well be synergistic."

✳

Faith, Science, and Your Risk of Cardiovascular Disease

We know that religious faith protects people from depression and reduces the duration of the affliction in those who become depressed. Now a compelling body of scientific research shows that depression increases the risk and danger of cardiovascular disease. Therefore, it's only logical to conclude that we can mobilize the healing power of faith in the fight against our leading killers, heart disease and stroke.

Chapter Nine

*

Religious People May Have Stronger Immune Systems

Every winter, local health departments advise people to get their annual inoculations against the latest strain of influenza. Public service announcements in your newspaper probably note that flu shots are especially important for "the elderly and people with weakened immune systems." And that's about the only time that most of us think about our immune systems.

The Immune System: Our Defense Against Disease

Simply stated, the immune system is the body's defensive works. Yours has helped maintain your health since before you were born. You might picture the skin as the walls of the castle, the mucous membranes in your mouth and nasal passages as the moat, and the throngs of tiny, specialized cells as the little soldiers guarding the castle against attack.

The immune system defends us against invaders from outside, such as viruses, bacteria, fungi, and other microbes. And our immune response may also protect us by destroying microscopic tumors, often no more than a clump of cells whose DNA has gone awry—which the specialized scavengers of our inner defenses recognize as "foreign"—before these tumors can grow and send metastatic seeds elsewhere in the body.

Included in the immune system are organs such as the spleen and thymus and the lymph nodes located throughout the body. The lymphatic system, paralleling the major blood vessels, helps to "filter" the blood for microbes. Specialized white blood cells, lymphocytes and leukocytes, circulate through the body, seeking out foreign substances. Certain types of lymphocytes, the B-cells, produce immunoglobulins that attach themselves to germs and make them easier for other white cells to surround and destroy. Other lymphocytes that directly attack microbes or cancer cells are called or T-killer cells. All of this microscopic community exists within a complex chemical milieu of proteins and hormones that can enhance or interfere with immune response.

Religious Involvement and the Immune System

While our Duke University research team was investigating the connection between religious involvement and blood pressure, we undertook a separate major study on the possible relationship between religious activity and the immune system among the elderly.[1]

This was the first major investigation to attempt to identify and measure such a possible link. In this regard we were, indeed, explorers on the frontiers of medicine. But we were building on a solid foundation of earlier work when we began our multiyear immune system investigation in the mid-1980s.

As we've seen, published research had shown a clear association between religious involvement—particularly church attendance—and better physical health among the elderly.[2] Again, our Duke hypertension study showed that older people who both attended religious services and frequently prayed or studied the Bible were 40 percent less likely to have dangerously high diastolic blood pressure than their less religiously involved peers. And, of course, there was all the other research suggesting that frequent church attenders had lower rates of heart disease and stroke, survived longer with less disability, and enjoyed better emotional health than less frequent attenders.

My colleagues and I were intrigued by these findings. We spent hours in conference rooms, hunched over plastic cups of tepid coffee, debating the merits of reports that demonstrated the association between religious involvement and better health, particularly among people in later life. But attempting to explain this connection in exact scientific terms was not going to be easy.

Earlier research studies linking greater religious involvement with lower rates of depression (independent of emotional support from family and friends), we judged, pointed toward a psychological basis for the physical health benefits of regular religious involvement. Remember that chronic psychological stress and depression have consistently been associated with the release of fight-or-flight hormones such as cortisol and a variety of other substances our bodies produce under such emotional challenges. The long-term overproduction of these hormones has been connected to cardiovascular disease through well-understood biological pathways.

Depression, Stress Hormones, and the Immune System

But how do stress and depression affect the immune system? In the spring of 1992, my Duke University colleague Dr. Ranga Krishnan brought me a pioneering study that had just been published in the *Archives of General Psychiatry*.[3] Dr. Krishnan had been on a research team investigating whether the well-documented overproduction of stress hormones in depressed patients was associated with enlargement of the adrenal glands.

"We've found something rather interesting, Harold," Ranga said, laying his manuscript and several computed tomography (CT) scan printouts on my desk.

The team Dr. Krishnan worked with had studied thirty-eight patients with major depression. Using CT scans, the researchers found that twelve of the depressed people had obvious adrenal gland enlargement, indicative of chronic tissue swelling. The scans showed the volume of the adrenal glands in these depressed patients to be significantly larger than those of people free of depression.

"You can actually *see* the physiological impact of major depression," Krishnan added, tapping a pencil on the faint gray swirls of the radiology films.

Indeed, the adrenal cortex or outer shell of the glands in several scans was obviously distended. Although this particular type of physiological research was not my specialty, I began to grasp the implications of the pioneering study.

Cortisol is one of the principal stress hormones, the others being epinephrine and norepinephrine, all secreted by the adrenal glands. If depression could cause these glands to visibly swell, as displayed in Dr. Krishnan's CT scans, the overabundance of cortisol in people suffering this emotional illness might well have a long-term effect on their immune systems.

After all, it had been proven that cortisol suppressed immune function. This is why people receiving organ transplants are given heavy doses of cortisol-based medications, so that their immune systems will not reject the foreign heart, liver, or kidney tissue. And it was also well documented that the lifelong regimen of cortisol that transplant recipients needed to follow increased their vulnerability to infection.

Now Ranga Krishnan's team had documented that serious depression actually provoked enlargement, what doctors call "hypertrophy" of the very glands that produced cortisol in the human body.

Later research conducted at the University of California, Los Angeles, using more sensitive MRI scans, confirmed that depression caused adrenal gland enlargement. The UCLA team found that adrenal gland volume was significantly larger in depressed patients than in people free of depression. But the researchers found that the adrenal gland volume of depressed people could be reduced a dramatic 70 percent when these patients were successfully treated.[4]

We recognized that chronic emotional problems could weaken the immune system by impairing the effectiveness of immune cells like lymphocytes to defend against bacteria, viruses, or even tiny tumors. In general, evidence showed that long-term depressive disorders increased susceptibility to other disease.[5]

Obviously, the power of religious faith and practice both to protect people from depression and to help them recover if afflicted might have major implications on their physical health through this intriguing biological pathway.

*

The Pioneering Duke Study

This line of reasoning led us to explore whether religiously active people—as measured by their frequency of attendance at services—might have healthier immune systems than their less religiously active counterparts. Since religiously active persons coped better with stress and were less likely to be depressed, perhaps their immune systems might likewise be stronger.

Once more, we turned to people participating in the large Establishment of Populations for Epidemiologic Studies of the Elderly (EPESE) research project sponsored by the National Institutes of Health. In 1986, my team worked with researchers who had randomly selected 4,000 men and women living in North Carolina and age sixty-five and over. About half of the people were black and half white.

We interviewed the people every eighteen months, either by telephone or in person, for six years. Beyond standard data on age, gender, and race, we assessed their ability to perform the tasks of daily living and whether they had chronic physical illness, including heart problems, hypertension, diabetes, stroke, and cancer. We also screened them for depression and negative life events such as bereavement.

During interviews, we asked the participants the standard question we had earlier devised to assess their religious attendance (as a measure of religious involvement): "How often do you attend religious services or other religious meetings?" They had six possible responses ranging from "never/almost never" to "more than once a week."

In 1992, our team visited 1,718 surviving participants from the original study and drew blood for analysis.

Interleukin-6: Canary in the Mine Shaft

We needed reliable biological markers in order to compare the strength or weakness of the people's immune systems. So we selected as our principal indicator a protein called interleukin-6 (IL-6) that the body produces in response to inflammation and which performs an important role in our immune systems.

High IL-6 levels indicate a weakened immune system that is not functioning at optimum performance. For example, patients with AIDS have high blood levels of IL-6. Elevated IL-6 is also found in many older people and is thought to be connected to the fundamental aging process, including increased susceptibility to the diseases of the elderly: certain cancers, as well as Type II diabetes, rheumatoid arthritis, Alzheimer's disease, and post-menopausal osteoporosis. Research has shown that elevated IL-6 is also found among people with impaired ability to perform daily tasks or with cardiovascular disease.[6]

There is also some evidence that IL-6 level in the higher range detected in older people may be a predictor of future health problems. But so-called higher ranges are indeed so small they could have not even been detected twenty years ago. Our basic yardstick for measuring IL-6 was picograms per milliliter of blood (pg/ml); that's a *trillionth* of a gram in thousandths of a liter of serum. Research suggests that people with IL-6 levels greater than 5 pg/ml may have weakened immune systems.

Planning this multiyear study, we began to envision IL-6 levels as the canaries that miners used to carry down in the coal shafts as crude but effective early-warning devices on the buildup of invisible but deadly gases.

Healthy "Doses" of Religion

After analyzing the blood samples, we divided our subjects into two main groups—those with IL-6 levels less than and those with levels greater than 5 pg/ml—as an indicator of strong versus weakened immune systems. We chose older people for this first-ever study on the effect of religious involvement on immune status because the elderly are more vulnerable to problems with their immune systems due to the effects of aging and disease. Thus any potential impact of religious activity on immune function might be more easily discovered in older adults.

We were also interested in IL-6 because research had shown that psychological stress increases the level of this substance as well as other inflammatory cytokines. Depressed people often have higher levels of these chemicals circulating in their blood.

Rather than bet all our chips on IL-6, however, we elected to measure other markers in the blood that are linked to inflammatory and immune responses. These included a complex mix of obscure substances such as fibrin d-dimers (involved with coagulation at lesion or trauma sites), alpha-1, alpha-2, beta and gamma globulins, as well as lymphocytes and neutrophils, all of which regulate the immune and inflammatory responses in the body.

We spread the findings on IL-6 over a continuous scale from the lowest to the highest, and also separated out the people with the higher range (greater than 5 pg/ml). These same blood samples allowed us to check other indications of immune function or inflammation by measuring our alphabet soup of related substances and counting white blood cell lymphocytes, the microscopic "scavengers" often found in an immune system under stress.

Slightly more than one in ten of the participants (11.1 percent) had IL-6 levels greater than 5 pg/ml, indicating a weakened immune system.

We found that low religious attendance during the earlier period of the study did not prove to be a good predictor of high IL-6 levels six years later. So, we concluded from this evidence that any protective effect on the immune system probably came from current patterns of religious involvement, as opposed to past activity.

The findings were of great potential interest:

• People who frequently attended religious services in 1992, the year we took their blood for lab tests, were significantly less likely to have high IL-6 levels than their less religiously involved counterparts.
• Among those who never or rarely attended religious services in 1992, 15.7 percent had high IL-6 levels (greater than 5 pg/ml), indicating immune system problems.
• Among people who attended services once a week or more that year, however, only 8.8 percent had IL-6 levels greater than 5 pg/ml.
• Among those who attended services an intermediate degree (perhaps only twice a month or every few months), 11 percent had high IL-6 levels.

- This gradation from lowest IL-6 levels to highest shows what medical researchers call a "dose-effect" response with increasing religious activity.
- In 1992, of the 1,718 study participants, 957 were still attending church at least once a week, even though many were well into their eighties. Further, 873 (91.2 percent) of these religiously active people appeared to have healthy immune systems based on their levels of IL-6.
- In fact, those people who attended religious services to any degree were only about *one-half* as likely to have high IL-6 levels as nonattenders, even after we took into account other important demographic and physical health factors (such as age, race, gender, socioeconomic status, chronic illnesses, and disability level).
- Other indications of immune system health also seemed to be connected to religious involvement. For example, people who frequently attended services had lower levels of several important immune markers than their less religious peers. This relationship was present for four of the eight immune function tags we measured (alpha-2 globulin, lymphocytes, neutrophils, and high d-dimers).

As biomedical researchers, we found these results fascinating.

Older people who frequently attended religious services appeared to have stronger immune systems than those who did not.

However, we were even more surprised to learn there was no apparent connection between depression or negative life events and high levels of IL-6. These emotional factors also did not seem to influence the other immune system markers we measured.

The fact that we did not find any obvious connection between depression or negative life events in this relationship stumped our team for a while. Then we decided that the way we had measured depression, by self-rated symptoms, might not have identified people with levels of this affliction severe enough to weaken their immune systems. Likewise, measuring negative life events in the year prior to the study baseline in 1986 may have been too insensitive to determine the degree of stress that subjects were likely to be experiencing in 1992 when IL-6 levels were drawn.

Faith at the Cellular Level

Further, we thought that the relationship between frequent religious attendance and stronger immune systems might be a consequence of stress reduction not reflected by level of depression or negative circumstances. Perhaps regular religious participation enhances immune functioning by yet unknown mechanisms. These might include the feeling of belonging to a loving community or that intangible emotional warmth felt during intense worship and known as fellowship. Maybe the joyful experience of group worship (which in the Judeo-Christian tradition involves chanting and liturgical music) and the little-understood but profoundly moving state we call "adoration" might play a part in this intriguing relationship. Remember the flood of joy and inner peace that Dan experienced during Sabbath services at the synagogue when he was separated from his wife?

All of these elements of congregational worship evoke positive feelings that may counteract stress, perhaps even on the physiological level of our immune systems, and thus convey health effects that go far beyond simply preventing depression. So, the biomedical mechanism by which religious participation enhances immune functioning may still be stress-related, even if measurable depression or major life stress are not involved in the pathway.

We also wondered whether high IL-6 levels might produce lethargy that could have skewed our findings by preventing some people from attending religious service. But we found little evidence that this was the case. On the contrary, we learned to our surprise that people often made extraordinary efforts to continue worshiping with their congregations, despite advanced age and increasing disability (as Idler and Kasl had found in their Yale study).

This was a long and complicated study. But our entire team thought the hard work was well worth the effort. No previous published research had examined the relationship between religious participation and the immune system. We were able to demonstrate a consistent relationship between religious attendance and immune status, as seen through IL-6 levels and other biological indicators of immune function and inflammation. Although our findings, per se, do not *prove* that frequent religious attendance invariably leads to better physical health by strengthening the immune system, we believe the investigation has broken ground on an important frontier of medical research.

Therefore we were heartened when news of our findings sparked active interest among the news media. Local newspapers and television stations began lining up for interviews as soon as Duke University issued a press release on the study. Then I was deluged with interview requests from national magazines, newspapers, and radio and television networks. Finally, I began receiving calls at odd hours of the morning and night from the international news media in places like London, Hamburg, and Sydney.

But to me one of the most satisfying public comments on our years of hard work came from a respected colleague, Dr. Marcia Ory, a senior scientist at the National Institute on Aging. Noting that our study went far beyond anecdotal evidence on the relationship between religious involvement and good health, she told the Associated Press the research was "incredibly significant" because it investigated the "biological linkages" between religious involvement and the immune system. Then Dr. Ory added a compliment our entire team appreciates: "This is one of the pioneering studies."

The Implications

I believe that this research has far-reaching implications. First, even though our study investigated elderly people among whom it would have been normal to find widespread indications of weakened immune response—as shown by elevated IL-6 and inflammatory substance levels—many of the religiously involved seemed to have what we might call "younger" immune systems, based on their lower probability of having elevated IL-6 levels. This is certainly an aspect of the research that should be further investigated among *younger* participants. For example, the Alameda County study found generally better health among religiously involved adults twenty-one to sixty-five years old during their twenty-eight year follow-up. Yet we know life-threatening and disabling diseases such as Type II diabetes, rheumatoid arthritis, and several malignant cancers seem to be related to altered immune systems in younger adults. Will researchers find the same relationship between religious involvement and a healthier immune system in this age group? If so, the public health ramifications could be vast.

Faith and Cancer

Let's look back at the study Dr. Jeffrey Dwyer of the University of Florida conducted comparing religious denomination and cancer rates by county across America. Counties with the highest concentration of Mormons and conservative or moderate Protestants had the lowest rates, while counties with the highest proportion of liberal Protestants, Catholics, or Jews had the highest.

There are a number of possible explanations for this phenomenon. Conservative Protestants formed the great majority of the most religiously active people we investigated in our immune study. They often attend church both for long, emotionally fulfilling Sunday services and for evening worship during the week. These worship patterns are less pronounced among moderate and liberal Protestants. And in today's American Catholic church, frequency of attendance has dropped steadily. Sabbath synagogue worship among Jews has also been declining in recent decades, partially due to increasing interfaith marriages, in which neither spouse observes their original religion. Since the relationship between a weakened immune system and cancer has been suggested in several studies, it's intriguing to speculate that the impact of these falling rates of church and synagogue attendance on people's immune systems might be a factor in cancer rates. To me, this is certainly an area that should be investigated.

Many excellent research studies suggest a link between emotional health, including a sense of inner peace and well-being, and a stronger immune system, which may provide some level of protection against cancer. It is important to bear in mind that the "foot soldiers" of a healthy immune system—the specialized B and T lymphocytes—not only combat bacterial and viral infections, they attack and destroy ultratiny prototumors (theory of immune surveillance). Thus the immune system may play a vital role in protecting us from cancer. It's not surprising, therefore, that since the immune system naturally weakens with age, cancer is more prevalent among the elderly.

Stress, the Immune System, and Cancer

Dr. Alison Fife, a psychiatrist at Brigham and Women's Hospital in Boston, and her colleagues explored the historical background of research connecting emotional health, the immune system, and cancer.[7] After carefully evaluating over seventy major research investigations on this fascinating aspect of the mind-body connection, Dr. Fife's team concluded there was ample evidence that chronic psychological stress and emotional illness did indeed play a role in weakening the immune system, which in turn appeared to increase risk of thyroid disease, diabetes, cancer, and cardiovascular disorders.

"Stress is thought to depress the immune system and thus render an organism more susceptible to disease," the researchers noted, "especially those diseases closely linked with immune functioning, such as malignancy [cancer], infection, autoimmune disease, and allergy."

One of America's innovative cancer researchers, Dr. Barbara Andersen, recently began a team study of the relationship between psychological stress and immune response in women who'd had surgery for localized breast cancer.[8] The central questions the researchers were interested in concerned whether psychological stress plays a role in the progression of cancer and whether it is possible to reduce stress and slow tumor growth. Andersen's team observed that the stress of diagnosis and surgery for breast cancer can "affect the immune system, possibly reducing the ability of individuals with cancer to resist disease progression and metastatic spread." The researchers began their study with 116 women who'd undergone breast cancer surgery, assessing their immune responses by measuring levels of specialized "natural killer" (NK) and T-lymphocyte cells. Eventually, Andersen's study at Ohio State University will involve 235 breast cancer patients who will be divided into two groups. One will attend support groups for a year that emphasize emotional support and coping strategies designed to reduce stress. The health outcomes of these patients will be studied for several years.

Among the initial participants, the findings are already quite compelling. The team consistently found during repeated blood tests that higher stress levels significantly predicted a weakened ability of NK cells to surround and destroy foreign cells (like tumor cells or microbes), indicating a disrupted immune system. Higher stress levels also significantly predicted diminished response of these NK cells to an immune system modulator (gamma interferon), which can help activate the killer cells to destroy cancer cells. Further, stress was a consistent factor in reducing the effectiveness of blood lymphocytes, including lowering T-cell responsiveness, vital in controlling the spread of cancer.

Dr. Andersen's team found interesting the mounting evidence suggesting that "stress reduction interventions may *enhance* certain aspects of the cellular immune response," so important in preventing the spread of cancer from the original tumor site.

In many ways, these initial findings bolster the evidence we discovered at Duke during our immune study. Breaking the grip of stress through intense counseling—or through frequent emotionally bolstering religious involvement—may help strengthen our immune systems, especially as we age.

Body, Soul & Spirit

I believe it's significant that increasing numbers of doctors involved with cancer therapy are beginning to recognize the healing power of faith. Recently, the Cancer Treatment Centers of America, which operate at hospitals nationwide, began offering patients a program called Body, Soul & Spirit as part of their comprehensive therapy. This is spiritual counseling meant to augment traditional support groups that supplement surgery, chemotherapy and other medical treatment, and therapeutic radiation.

In the program, counselors work with the patients, their families, and loved ones to offer a variety of spiritual services. These include individual or group prayer, meeting with a faith counselor of the patient's choice, weekly religious and Communion services, and support groups that focus on healing, faith, and the positive aspects of life.

Kurt Walbrandt, an executive with the organization, calls the pastoral healing program a "vital component to our 'total person' approach to care." He agrees that both the prevention of depression and the strengthening of the immune system that such spiritually directed counseling might provide can bolster a patient's resolve to fight the illness.

Although there is a pressing need for extensive research on the biological pathways involved with longer survival following social support sessions among cancer patients, there already exists convincing evidence that this type of counseling, which helps people face and deal with fears of dying—the essence of the Cancer Treatment Centers' spiritual counseling program—is helpful.

A research team led by Dr. David Spiegel of Stanford University conducted a ten-year follow-up of breast cancer patients, half of whom received routine care, the other active psychosocial intervention. There was a significant increase in average survival time—36.6 months for the psychosocial treatment group versus 18.9 months for the others.[9] Unfortunately, researchers did not examine if these women's immune systems were involved in this increased survival.

But it would be fascinating to compare the immune systems of cancer patients undergoing the Body, Soul & Spirit counseling with the systems of those who do not.

＊

Bereavement and the Immune System

Research led by Holly G. Prigerson, Ph.D., of the University of Pittsburgh School of Medicine, focused on traumatic grief as a risk factor for contracting mental and physical disease.[10] Her team studied 150 women and men whose husbands and wives were terminally ill. Once their spouses died, a significant number of these people were so traumatized that they developed severe emotional problems. The existence of symptoms of psychiatric disorder among widows and widowers six months after bereavement, the researchers found, could actually predict increased incidence of illnesses such as cancer, cardiovascular disease, suicidal depression, and severe eating disorders over the next two years.

The researchers discovered that the total risk of developing cancer was "significantly higher" among the study participants undergoing traumatic grief than among those who were not.

Other studies have suggested a connection between losing a husband or wife and weakened immune response. In 1983, Dr. Steven Schleifer, from Mount Sinai School of Medicine in New York, and his colleagues found a "highly significant suppression" of lymphocytes in the immune system among men whose wives had just died of cancer.[11] The researchers speculated that many of the thousands of deaths that occur among widows and widowers in their first year of bereavement might be related to weakened immune response. This study follows similar research on reduced T- and B-cell counts indicative of weakened immune response among bereaved spouses in Australia in the 1970s.[12]

But the emotional succor of religious faith and membership in a supporting congregation may help prevent such traumatic grief. First, all Judeo-Christian denominations draw on emotionally evocative liturgy during the final days of life, death, and interment. The last rites of the Roman Catholic Church evolved from earlier Jewish practices of anointing the dead and preparing their earthly remains for burial. Music plays a significant role in most funeral services. And, among the faithful, the firm belief that the beloved member of the family and congregation has passed on to a better place eases the emotional burden on the survivors.

Rebounding from Bereavement

The ability of religiously involved people to rebound both physically and emotionally from bereavement, without succumbing to traumatic grief, is worth reexamining.

We only have to look at the emotional strength Louise Hudson drew from her abiding religious faith following the death of her husband, Walter, to understand how religion shields people from the traumatic impact of bereavement.

Paul Burns also suffered a type of severe bereavement when he was finally forced to recognize that his wife and lifelong partner, Lorene, had been taken from him by the cruel affliction of Alzheimer's disease. Although he had lost the multidimensioned and loving person Lorene was, Paul has actually gained something from the emotional pain of this bereavement by discovering a rich vein of spirituality within himself.

It might be coincidental, but neither Louise nor Paul has suffered from the afflictions of the elderly related to a weakened immune system.

The Healing Essence of Congregational Worship

During the media blitz that followed the publication of the Duke immune study in December 1997, a number of reporters seemed curious if this research somehow "proved" the existence of a divine power that intervened to protect the health of the faithful. As a scientist, of course, I had to answer no. That certainly was not the intention of this investigation. This type of question touches on the dilemma of a researcher studying the relationship between religion and health.

"We're not trying to prove that there is a higher power," I told one

reporter. "But maybe believing in that higher power could be an important key to people's health." Whatever the interpretation some of the
American and overseas reporters wanted to place on our research, I emphasized that what the investigation revealed was that the immune systems of people actively involved in their religious community were
simply "functioning better."

It is going to take years of additional research before we can pin
down with scientific certainty the exact biological pathways apparently
linking religious involvement, a strong immune system, and improved
health.

But it might be helpful to compare the religious lives and the health
of some of the people whom we've encountered so far in this book.

Obviously, Khalita Jones, the brave young university student fighting her long battle against the severe autoimmune disorder aplastic
anemia, is a person whose life literally depends on the resilience of her
immune system. She is constantly at risk of contracting infections from
common microbes that are harmless to people with normal immune response. As she struggles to balance the burden of her illness and the demands of her university classes, Khalita must walk a narrow line
between overextending herself physically and surrendering to unproductive lethargy.

Her doctors at the Duke University Medical Center continually
monitor her immune response, particularly the levels and activity patterns of specialized white blood cells and lymphocytes. Last spring, her
medical care team was at a loss to explain a series of blood tests that
showed her immune system had rebounded dramatically.

"I've been blessed," Khalita told one physician. "Not only do I have
a wonderful congregation here in Durham, but the people at my home
church are constantly praying for me."

Can Prayer Heal?

Indeed, Khalita Jones is acutely aware that the devout congregation at
her AME Zion church in Lexington, North Carolina, conducts a regu

lar prayer vigil, week in, week out, for her health. There is no direct *scientific* evidence that these "intercessory" prayers strengthen Khalita's immune system. The classic study on intercessory prayer was conducted by Dr. Randolph Byrd, a cardiologist in the institution at which I was a medical student and met Lee Daugherty, San Francisco General Hospital. Byrd randomly divided heart patients into two groups for a ten-month study. One group of 192 patients received intercessory prayer from a group of ministers and laypeople directing their supplications to the Judeo-Christian God. The control group of 201 patients received no such prayer. Knowledge of who was and who was not receiving prayer was strictly controlled.

All the patients were carefully screened for the progress of their heart disease and their response to medication and other therapy in the coronary care unit. The results were highly provocative. The heart patients who were prayed for suffered significantly fewer complications than those who received no prayer. Patients who were prayed for were five times less likely to require antibiotics for infections (a sign of good immune response), two and a half times less likely to suffer congestive heart failure, and had a significantly lower risk of sudden cardiac arrest.

Since then other institutions have been unable to replicate the findings of the Byrd study. However, Harvard Medical School's Herbert Benson is soon due to begin a much larger and longer similar intercessory prayer study, which will help settle the important question: whether the benefits of intercessory prayer can be demonstrated in a scientific manner.

One Aspect of Intercessory Prayer

How does this apply to Khalita Jones? First, Khalita knows she is the constant recipient of intercessory prayer, and that knowledge can affect her health by strengthening her psychologically, rather than by miraculous or supernatural means that medical science cannot explore. She describes the profound comfort she receives from this knowledge as helping her build inner "strength." For a person with her illness, such strength—as opposed to the feverish debilitation and pains of chronic infection—might well indicate a strengthened immune response. Second, Khalita connects her own daily spiritual discipline of prayer and scripture reading to the larger efforts of her two congregations. In other words, she is an *active* participant in her quest for recovery.

The Oxman Study

This brings to mind the classic Dartmouth University study of cardiac surgery patients led by Dr. Thomas Oxman. You'll recall that among the 232 patients he studied for five months after their open-heart surgery, none of the 37 people who described themselves as "deeply religious" died. And only 5 percent of those who attended church at least every few months died in the six months following their operations, compared with 12 percent of those who attended rarely or never.

It stands to reason that the religiously involved people Oxman studied were not praying in a vacuum, but rather as part of a faith community. Once more, did patients' knowledge that a body of the faithful had banded together in supplication with them somehow enable them to marshal inner reserves of physical strength to help bring about healing? These are vitally important questions for the medical profession.

Loving Kindness

Whatever the pathways involved, Khalita Jones does in fact receive emotional and physical strength from attendance at religious services. At her home AME church in Lexington, North Carolina, Khalita regularly experiences the intense joy of robust African-American worship, during which services can last for hours. Fervent gospels and testimonials from members of the congregation alternate with deeply rhythmic and moving music. For Khalita, attending these services is virtually a renewing experience. She feels transported past the physical confines of her afflicted body when she is surrounded by her family and the loving bonds of church members she has known since infancy. This was the type of "belonging" I had in mind when I commented in our immune study that regular attendance at religious services may convey health effects that transcend the simple prevention of depression.

In Durham, the members of the racially diverse university community church Khalita attends provide another type of support. Although they intervene to help Khalita with daily tasks when necessary, they constantly guide her toward physical independence. They truly see Khalita Jones as their sister who needs temporary assistance. Helping her with shopping or bringing her meals when she is too sick to cook is not an imposition; they would quite naturally do the same for any family member. And Khalita understands that she is a member of their family. This type of unconditional spiritual love, which some theologians have called *agape*, dates back millennia to the roots of the Judeo-Christian heritage. When Jesus of Nazareth preached charity toward the poor and afflicted, he was echoing the Jewish tradition of *Gemilut Chasadim* (acts of loving kindness). Khalita Jones and millions of other members of caring congregations respond to such love.

The devout certainty of Khalita and her congregation that God does intervene directly in people's lives bolsters her confidence that there are profound spiritual reasons why she has been chosen to undergo the long physical ordeal of her illness. This allows Khalita to pray with a calm intensity that banishes stress that might have built up from the pain and uncertainty of her condition.

Khalita has called herself a "joyful person," describing a state of inner tranquillity that may have virtually helped keep her alive years longer than a standard medical prognosis would have indicated.

A Lifetime of Healthy Faith

When Messiah Evangelical Lutheran Church preschool teacher Helen Koebert, now eighty-two, describes her health, she often chuckles. "The doctors never saw too much of me."

In fact, neither Helen nor her sisters Lorraine Kummers and Esther

Hart have suffered premature illness. Helen can't remember the last time she had a cold or the flu, a good indication of a strong immune system.

They have been lifelong members of their church in Milwaukee. But their involvement surpasses mere attendance, what might be considered "extrinsic" religiosity, as we defined it earlier. Over seventy-five years, the three sisters have volunteered to transform the unassuming church building into a sacred structure, not through architectural innovation or works of art, but through loving acts of labor. Both in the original modest clapboard structure on the corner of Kinnickinnic and Fernwood Avenues and in the larger nearby modern church, Helen and her sisters have washed and carefully ironed altar cloths and polished candelabra and sacramental silver.

Their connection to the church and its congregation runs deep. As with Khalita Jones, the Messiah faith community is an extended family for the sisters. They were baptized and married in the church, and they know their funerals will be held there. Their profound attachment, as manifested through their volunteer work as preschool teachers, is in fact an act of loving kindness that dates from the foundations of the Judeo-Christian religious tradition.

Again, I believe scientists could design serious research projects investigating the physiological pathways involved in the benefits such devout and religiously active people derive from living their faith.

A Case for Protective Faith?

One interesting study was led by Haitung King and published in the *Journal of the National Cancer Institute* in 1980. The researchers compared mortality rates from several diseases, including certain cancers, among almost 30,000 American clergymen from predominantly white denominations with the rates in a similar number of lay peers. Standard statistical probability predicted that 7,243 of these clergymen would have died during the ten years of the study period. But only 5,207 died. This 28 percent differential was attributed to a substantially lower risk of lung, stomach, bladder, and rectal cancers. But the clergymen also had dramatically lower death rates from cardiovascular and kidney disease than their layman counterparts.

Intriguingly, the strongest protective benefits came at younger ages. This suggests that not only were the clergymen leading a healthier lifestyle (reduced smoking and alcohol use) than their secular counterparts, but they might have also received some intangible benefit from their faith and religious involvement—perhaps through prayer and worship, or regular religious giving.[13]

Heart Health and the Immune Response

If so, this might partially explain the lower rates of cardiovascular disease that repeated studies have found among religiously active people. There is a growing body of thought in contemporary medicine—some call it a paradigm shift—that coronary heart disease may be initially caused by a virus. Researchers at the National Institutes of Health and a separate team at Johns Hopkins School of Public Health have found increasing evidence that infections from the common cytomegalovirus (CMV), a garden-variety member of the diverse strain of herpes virus, can damage coronary arteries, producing the original lesion around which vascular blockages develop and eventually lead to heart attack.

In people with healthy immune systems, the cytomegalovirus is likely to be kept in check. But, researchers suggest, for some individuals the virus can lead to recurrent arterial blockage. Dr. Stephen E. Epstein, chief of cardiology at the National Heart, Lung, and Blood Institute, was on one team that published results on the viral–coronary artery disease link in the *New England Journal of Medicine*.[14] An important finding of the study, Epstein suggests, is that "prior infection with CMV is a strong independent risk factor" for arterial blockages occurring after plaque-clearing surgical procedures. Dr. F. Javier Nieto and researchers from Johns Hopkins found even stronger evidence of an association between CMV and coronary artery disease.[15]

It would be interesting to conduct research on devoutly religious people who have overcome heart disease, such as Louise Hudson, to determine how their immune systems handle CMV.

Faith, AIDS, and the Immune System

When Bill Maceri, the young artist who contracted AIDS in Berlin, returned to New York, his immune system was devastated. Like many AIDS patients, Bill was plagued by opportunistic infections that attacked his respiratory and gastrointestinal systems. It's well to remember that HIV, the microbe that causes AIDS, is the human immuno*deficiency* virus, which by definition destroys immunity. One of the most alarming signs of Bill's severely deficient immunity was the count of his T-lymphocytes, and T-helper cells.

"My T-cells were down around zero when I was stuck alone in that dismal studio out in Bedford-Stuyvesant," Bill recalls.

After Bill began his spiritual quest, however, and before he started on lifesaving combined therapy with the new protease inhibitors, his immune system had already begun to respond. Using traditional devotional prayer focusing on the Holy Trinity of his Roman Catholic upbringing, as well as on a less-defined benevolent providence, Bill was able to reduce his anxiety levels and gain improved inner calm.

Once he began the new medication therapy, Bill intensified his spiritual practices. Prayer—both traditional and non-conventional—became an important part of his daily life. Reading the inspirational book *Conversations with God* by Neale Donald Walsh convinced Bill Maceri that he could speak directly to God because, as a suffering human and a part of divine creation, there was no barrier between his own finite physical life and God's infinite presence.

Today, through a combination of medication, prayer, other spiritual practices, and strong support from family and friends, Bill Maceri's immune system is much healthier.

The strengthening of Bill's AIDS-ravaged immune response does not appear to be a fluke. Teresa E. Woods, a psychology researcher at the University of Miami in Coral Gables, Florida, recently led a study on the relationship between religion, depression, and immune status among gay men infected with HIV.[16] The team investigated two distinct aspects of faith among 106 gay men who had tested positive for HIV and had shown some symptoms. These aspects were religious coping (putting trust in God, seek God's help, etc.) and religious practices (religious attendance, frequency of prayer, spiritual discussions, and reading scripture or devotional material). The men were then tested for depression and the status of their immune systems were assessed by measuring T-helper-inducer cells (CD4+).

The results were interesting, and supported our finding that religious involvement may strengthen the immune system. Religious coping was significantly associated with lower scores on a standard test for depression, but had no significant separate connection to specific immune system markers.

Conversely, men more involved in religious practices such as attendance at services, prayer, and scripture reading had higher CD4+ cell counts and percentages. But these religious practices as separate factors did not seem to affect their levels of depression or anxiety.

The Miami researchers carefully took into account relevant health issues, including the diagnosed progression of HIV-related illness or AIDS and any medication regimens the men were following.

Even after taking these factors into account, the relationships between religious coping and lower depression, and religious practices and higher CD4+ counts persisted. The findings suggest that religiosity may be an important resource for maintaining optimal mental health and immune system functioning among men with HIV infection.

Magic Johnson's Miracle

It's interesting to note that the person who is probably the most famous HIV-infected individual in the world, NBA legend Earvin "Magic" Johnson, firmly agrees that religious faith and practice play a leading role in preserving his health. Since contracting the virus, Magic

Johnson has become intensely religious. Being able to maintain his strength and active involvement in entreprenurial endeavors in America's blighted inner cities is proof, Johnson says, that he is living a "miracle." He knows, however, that the virus still lurks in the confines of his body, kept at bay through a combination of advanced medicine and timeless faith. "I'm not cured," Magic Johnson recently commented. "But I am healed."

Chapter Ten

Religious People Use Fewer Expensive Hospital Services

A Health Care Crisis

Most of us realize that there's a health care crisis looming in our future. In America alone, the Baby Boom generation of seventy-seven million people is passing through middle age and will enter retirement and later life in the twenty-first century. Over the next forty years, this generation will add fifty million people to the Medicare rolls. Many experts predict that this aging of our population will eventually stretch health resources beyond their limits.

We can see clear signs of this emerging problem today. Between 1980 and 1997, the Medicare budget exploded to over $200 billion, even though our elderly population increased by only six million people. Yet the total cost of medical services in America is already immense: In the year 2007, about one-fifth of our economy—a staggering two *trillion* dollars—will be devoted to health care.

And all of us recognize that advances in medicine, ranging from open-heart surgery to kidney dialysis to new cancer treatments, combined with almost universal government or private health insurance have extended the lives of older Americans. These developments are bound to increase the number of people suffering chronic illnesses such as heart disease and cancer and physical disability due to stroke and osteoporosis. Today there are only about two million severely disabled older Americans, but the level of serious disability is projected to rise as high as twelve million in the next fifty years.[1]

All of us in the medical professions accept that something is going to have to give on the cost-containment front. We hope that quality of care won't suffer, but that may well be the case. Today, more than 70 percent of Americans belong to some form of managed care, often corporately owned health maintenance organizations (HMOs). Although they are generally dedicated to providing excellent care, HMOs must also produce a reasonable rate of return for their investors. Otherwise, they'll go out of business. So HMOs, in particular, are going to be squeezed financially as the Baby Boom turns gray.

People naturally suffer more illness as they age. This leads to the incredible—and steadily mounting—cost of treating older patients in the hospital. On the average, people over age sixty are hospitalized twice as often as younger adults and account for almost 50 percent of all short hospital stays. And by far, treatment—ranging from surgery to psychotherapy—in a modern hospital, with its extensive laboratories, operating rooms, and computerized MRI and CT imaging suites, is the single most expensive aspect of medical care.

Fortunately, most of us go through life spending just a few days as hospital patients. But then, in our final years, we begin to accumulate days and even weeks as hospitalized patients receiving expensive services, often from multiple departments, which we call "acute care." Our total cost of lifelong treatment soars. A recent article in the medical journal The Lancet showed that total health care costs for people age fifty and older rise "exponentially" by age until the end of life.[2]

Beyond this financial burden, hospitalized acute care patients also often suffer isolation and anguish. A modern hospital room, with its banks of beeping and blinking equipment, can depersonalize a seriously ill person. All too often, the "heroic" life-extending measures involving mechanical respirators and feeding tubes, which became increasingly commonplace in the 1980s, have the ironic effect of prolonging physical existence while crushing patients' unique personalities and their spirits.

As a gerontologist, I recognized long ago that one of medicine's primary goals should be to search for ways to reduce the need for hospitalization among older people. Certainly preventive practices, wider disease screening, wellness monitoring, as well as better habits of nutrition and exercise, would all play a role in keeping the lid on health care costs as people age. But the single biggest saving would be to curtail the number and length of hospital stays. Could reducing the need for acute care hospitalization be a practical goal, I wondered, given prevailing medical ethics and legal considerations?

Large, well-designed research studies conducted at Duke University and other institutions have clearly demonstrated a connection between religious involvement and better health, especially in later life. And better health should be reflected in fewer, shorter admissions to hospitals among acute care patients.

My colleague Dr. David B. Larson and I decided to investigate this intriguing theory in 1993. Larson, a psychiatrist with an advanced degree in public health science, is president of the National Institute for Healthcare Research. Over the years, he has assembled voluminous research showing that religious faith and involvement are widespread among Americans. He aptly described religion as the "forgotten factor" in much of the traditional research examining the psychological and social influences on health.

Working with David Larson, I found there was a particular lack of information on how religious faith and activities affect hospital-use patterns among older people. To ignore religion as an influence on older Americans' health seemed to us ridiculous. After all, recent Gallup polls showed that 96 percent of Americans believed in God or a universal spirit, and religious faith and practice among people over age sixty-five was even more intense: 98 percent of these elderly believe in God; 95 percent pray; and 53 percent attend religious service weekly or more often.

Further, I had seen in some of my earliest research that significant numbers of older people not only rely on their religious faith and on practices such as prayer to help maintain their health or alleviate problems, but also turn to their faith to cope with the stress caused by physical illness.

These and other studies had led public health researchers to suggest that religion might play a role in how often a person needed general medical services. Almost twenty-five years ago, pioneering researcher David Mechanic, Ph.D., of the department of sociology at the University of Wisconsin, Madison, showed clear evidence that people's religious background could have a significant influence on the patterns of illness they suffered and the types of medical services they might need.

In one of my first studies on the impact of depression on the outcome of medical illness, my team showed that older people with physical illness who were also depressed spent about twice as long in the hospital as their nondepressed fellow patients. If religious persons coped better with physical illness and suffered less depression, then perhaps their hospital stays might also be shorter.

Even with this body of evidence, David Larson and I were surprised to find there had been almost no research examining the connection between the religious faith or affiliation of older people and their need for hospital care due to physical illnesses. One small study published in 1990 of elderly women hospitalized with hip fractures found that their degree of religiousness predicted a greater distance they could walk at discharge compared with less religious women, but the research did not investigate the effect of religion on length of hospital stay.

When we conducted an extensive database search, Larson and I found that our research team at Duke was one of the few groups investigating this relationship, and the only group to study this among the elderly.[3] But the thrust of that study was on the use of religion as a coping mechanism (emotional dependence on religion to ease psychological stress) and not primarily on length of hospital stay. We had not been able to find a relationship between religious coping and days hospitalized, possibly because people did not turn to religion for comfort until they found themselves in a hospital with a severe illness. This would disguise any positive effects of religious involvement on the need for acute hospital care.

Hospitalization and Religious Commitment

So David Larson and I decided to expand a larger ongoing project examining the effect of depression on the use of health services among hospitalized older patients to determine whether religious involvement and affiliation had an impact on the length of their hospital stays. For our study group, we chose a consecutive series of patients age sixty or over admitted to the general medicine, cardiology, and neurology inpatient services of Duke University Medical Center beginning in August 1993. We eventually registered and interviewed 542 men and women, with an average age of just over seventy.[4]

We wanted to test several hypotheses:

- First, we believed high attendance at religious services would be associated with lower rates of acute hospital care during the year prior to their admission at Duke, and also with a shorter stay during that hospitalization.
- We also believed that the older patients not affiliated with religious organizations would have used more hospital services during the prior year and would have had longer stays.
- Finally, we believed that any apparent health benefit of religious involvement and affiliation would persist even after we statistically took into account factors likely to affect length of hospital stay, such as age, sex, race, and severity of illness and degree of disability. We also collected detailed information on the patients' family and social support networks and their level of depression.

During personal interviews, we asked our standard religious attendance question: "How often do you attend church or other religious meetings?" Patients could respond with six options ranging from "never" to "more than once a week." To determine religious affiliation, we asked the patients to choose from a list of fifty-seven different denominations, ranging from none through conservative and mainline Protestants, to Jewish and Catholic, to fundamentalist and Pentecostal.

We also asked how frequently and for how many days the patients had been hospitalized prior to their current admission at Duke, during both the previous year and the three prior months.

The complete body of data was carefully analyzed using rigorous computer models to compare all the possible variables, including number of hospital admissions and lengths of stays in the previous year and while at Duke, with religious attendance and affiliation. We carefully took into account the effects of age, sex, race, education, physical and emotional health, and levels of social support.

Once more, our findings were provocative and, we believe, important.

The probability of being hospitalized at least once in the previous year was a *substantial 56 percent lower* for those who attended church at least once per week ("frequent attenders") than for those who attended less frequently. Number of days hospitalized in both the previous year and the prior three months were also significantly lower among frequent attenders.

The length of hospital stay at Duke during the study was significantly lower among the religiously involved people than among their counterparts.

We also found that patients not affiliated with any religious denomination had significantly more hospital admissions in the previous year and tended to have spent more days in the hospital during the three months prior to their admission at Duke.

Our main findings were indeed significant:

- After we took into account all the variables, including medical illness, psychological health, support from family and friends, age, education, and race, we found that the people who attended church at least once a week *were 43 percent less likely* to have been admitted to the hospital in the prior year than the less religious participants.
- And the frequent attenders spent fewer days in the hospital in that year than the less religiously involved.
- Further, compared with patients affiliated with a religious denomination, those with no religious affiliation spent an average of *fourteen more days* at Duke University Medical Center (24.8 vs. 10.6 days) during their current hospital stay.
- That means that the religiously active people belonging to a faith community stayed less than *half* as long in the hospital as

people their own age and background, suffering similar illnesses, who lacked a denomination or membership in a congregation at which they regularly attended worship service.

To fully grasp the economic significance of our study, consider that the cost of hospitalization at Duke University Medical Center can be as high as $4,000 a *day*. This daily cost is similar to that at many other large teaching hospitals nationwide.

If having strong religious faith and frequently attending services can reduce an average hospital stay for an elderly patient by as much as fourteen days, as our research suggests, the per-patient saving might be as high as several hundred thousand dollars over the course of their later lives. Now multiply that by the seventy-seven million Baby Boomers who are approaching their elderly years. As I've often said, religious faith deals with the intangibles of the supernatural. But you can measure the practical benefits of religious faith to our beleaguered health care system in down-to-earth dollars.

To David Larson and me, accounting for the substantial differences in number of hospitalizations and lengths of stays between the religiously active and the noninvolved was a fascinating problem. Admission to a hospital these days is not an easy matter. A person has to show signs or symptoms of a fairly serious illness to be admitted. But once you have gone through all the paperwork and become an inpatient "case," there usually has to be some clear improvement in your condition before you are discharged. Yet the religiously active older patients we studied were being discharged on the average of fourteen days earlier than the people who seemed to lack religious involvement.

What was going on?

First, we found that many of our most religious participants were discharged following major surgery or serious medical illness after stays of only five or six days. For elderly patients, this pace of recovery was dramatic. David and I thought long and hard of what processes could lie behind this. Then I began to carefully read the comments on religion these patients had provided our interviewers. Obviously, strength of faith played a significant role in their healing.

One man, a sixty-five-year-old factory worker, was depressed before undergoing open-heart surgery. But during his talk with our interviewer, he spoke movingly about how he had "relied on the Lord" his entire life. He was discharged improved after only six days.

A woman of eighty with unstable angina remained alert and happy throughout her treatment. "The Lord always comforts me," she told our interviewer, adding that reading the Bible calmed her fears. She walked out of the hospital after only four days.

One retired government worker, a man in his early seventies, was hospitalized with dangerous vascular blood clots in both legs. During his interview he spoke expansively of his home congregation: "Church helps me deal with the stress of these medical problems," he stated. "I've always depended on a higher power to see me through." He responded well to treatment and was discharged after five days.

One quiet old man had been hospitalized because of fainting spells related to congestive heart problems. When he spoke to our interviewer about his religious faith, his eyes filled with tears of joy. "Christ strengthens me. I know my eternity is sealed, so nothing on this earth can harm me." Despite his serious problems on admission, he was discharged in good condition only five days later.

Michael Walsh, sixty-three, a veterinarian with a busy practice, had been admitted to Duke Hospital following severe shortness of breath after he'd been lifting heavy bags at his clinic. Cardiologists diagnosed him with atrial fibrillation, a potentially life-threatening rhythm problem in the heart's upper chambers. Certainly anxiety and stress can worsen this condition. But our interviewer found Walsh serene, projecting an almost jovial tranquillity. "I certainly wasn't always that way," Dr. Walsh recalls. "For years, I'd been anxious and stressed out, sweating every little detail in my work and daily life. I smoked and drank too much." But at Alcoholics Anonymous meetings he'd learned to take control over the inner fears that had long ruled his life. He'd been impressed by AA's emphasis on finding personal tranquillity "through prayer and meditation to improve our conscious contact with God." Michael Walsh became active again in the Catholic faith of his childhood. When he was admitted to Duke with his heart problems, he told our team that his guiding principle in times of trouble had become, "Let go, and let God." Dr. Walsh was discharged after an admission of only four days.

David Larson and I agreed that these strong testaments of faith suggested that the patients experienced less stress and drew deep inner comfort from their religion. Beyond these people's use of religion to cope with the immediate emotional stress of their illness and hospitalization, their status as frequent attenders meant they were also active members of a supportive faith community. We only have to think of Frank Kozoman, Khalita Jones, and Rachel Cowan to recognize the emotional strength people derive from such a congregation during times of crisis.

Protection from depression that the religiously active often enjoy might have been a factor in their shorter hospital stays. It was, of course, also possible that belonging to a caring faith community meant that these frequent attenders were more likely to have their health problems diagnosed earlier and treated more effectively, thus decreasing their need for hospitalization.

Personally, I tend to think that a number of factors are involved, including stress reduction and the less easily quantifiable benefits of religious involvement on cardiovascular health and on strengthening the immune system.

Certainly people are not discharged only four or five days of hospitalization if they suffer dangerous high blood pressure, increased clotting risk, and a debased immune system that leaves them vulnerable to infection. I'm definitely not suggesting that modern medicine, with its amazing surgical techniques and miracle drugs, does not play a major role in recovery. But in our study, almost everyone received similar levels of medical treatment. Yet the fact remains that a significant number of religiously active people were discharged from the hospital an average of fourteen days earlier than people their own age with similar illness who were not religiously involved.

Whatever the processes at work, I think it's vital that other researchers try to replicate our study, especially outside the Bible Belt, where religion plays such an active role in people's lives.

Once more, I'm a physician researcher, not an evangelist. So it's clearly premature to suggest that elderly people—including the millions of Baby Boomers who are soon to become elderly—rush out and join a religious congregation the way they dash to the nutrition store in the mall to stock up on the latest Asian herbal remedy. Based on our study, it's also too early to suggest that the mammoth health insurance industry grant people who frequently attend church lower premium rates.

But what David Larson and I *are* suggesting is that, given the inevitable burden of health care costs of our aging population, and in view of the relationship that we and others have found between religious involvement and the use of terribly expensive hospital services, public health experts should take a much closer look at the healing power of faith. And people who have neglected their spiritual side because of the demands of a busy life might do well to give themselves time to reassess their priorities. This suggestion is especially relevant because faith communities such as churches and synagogues are widely available, and involvement in them costs people and government virtually nothing when compared with hospital care.

Dr. Elisabeth McSherry, Pioneer in the Pastoral Care Revolution

Almost twenty years ago, Elisabeth McSherry, M.D., a former professor of clinical pediatrics at the University of California, San Francisco, began investigating the economic and scientific basis for establishing closer links between traditional and "whole person" medicine, which includes the spiritual side of our lives. To explore this fascinating area, Dr. McSherry went to work for the Veterans Administration as a cost-effectiveness expert in Massachusetts. She devoted years researching an intriguing question: Could devoting more attention to people's spiritual needs when they are ill lead to better outcomes in their physical and emotional health and thus reduce the cost of health care and make better use of increasingly scarce resources?

One of Dr. McSherry's first important findings was that there were, indeed, medical and psychological reasons for the healing professions to treat both the body and spirit.[5] Dr. McSherry reviewed scores of studies confirming that the American population was highly religious and that the majority of people were deeply interested in the "spiritual aspect" of their lives, which touched on transcendental issues such as ultimate meaning, purpose, and values. People often pondered these difficult questions during times of stress caused by physical illness in themselves or a loved one. Yet she also found that fifty years of modern scientific Western medicine had largely ignored the spiritual side of life. In other words, Elisabeth McSherry was one of the leaders on this medical frontier where the body, the mind, and the transcendental dimensions of the spirit intersect.

She correctly predicted that hospices would fill an increasingly important role for Americans who wish to pass through the final phases of terminal illness surrounded by their loved ones and clergy in a warmer atmosphere than a typical modern hospital room usually provides. Dr. McSherry also foresaw the growing importance of pastoral psychotherapy counseling, in which mental health professionals—in a reversal of Freud's earlier criticism of religion—would tend to people's spiritual lives to help bolster their emotional health.

Even in the early 1980s when she began her research, Dr. McSherry suggested that scientific researchers such as myself would be able to quantify the tangible benefits accruing from "spiritual health care." She was, in fact, predicting the emergence of the important distinction between "healing" and "cure" that we have stressed throughout this book.

There were practical aspects to the work of Dr. McSherry and her research colleagues. As modern hospitals took form over the past thirty years, evolving into the often impersonal large regional medical centers of today, McSherry envisioned an increasingly activist role for pastoral care specialists, including clergy from the patient's congregation, hospital staff chaplains, and lay spiritual-care volunteers.

One of the depersonalizing elements for the hospitalized patient at modern medical centers, McSherry noted, was the almost industrial trend of "streamlining [care] production" into groups of patients with similar illnesses that became known as the "diagnosis-related group" (DRG). This process was both cost-effective for the hospital and optimized the use of skilled professionals in such fields as surgery or radiology.

But in building these efficient DRG treatment teams, Dr. McSherry aptly pointed out, pastoral care was usually neglected. This was not merely a question of loneliness or spiritual isolation. Rather, she emphasized, there was ample evidence that chaplain visits affected the physical health of the patient, and thus the cost to the hospital. One study from the University of Virginia Medical Center, for example, demonstrated that orthopedic injury patients who received chaplain visits required 66 percent less pain medication, made two-thirds fewer calls on the nursing staff, and were discharged two days earlier than patients with similar diagnoses who received no chaplain visits.

"Lengths of stay and resource utilization can be significantly lowered," McSherry's research team predicted, "if the spiritual issues are adequately dealt with."[6]

The Spiritual Profile Assessment

Elisabeth McSherry pushed for the full integration of the spiritual counselors she called "truly modern" hospital chaplains into the rapidly evolving, ultraefficient hospital care system. One of the tools she recommended the chaplains use was a standardized Spiritual Profile Assessment (SPA), a type of questionnaire that would help pastoral counselors understand an individual patient's religious strengths and areas of vulnerability. The purpose of obtaining this type of spiritual diagnosis was to help all the busy members of the care team understand the whole person, rather than treating the patient as simply a physical entity.[7]

She conducted one of her most impressive demonstrations of the tangible health benefits patients receive from regular spiritual counseling in a study for the Veterans Affairs health system. Beginning in 1990, she led a project to chart the impact of daily chaplain visits using "full spiritual dimension diagnostics," including the Spiritual Profile Assessment, on patients hospitalized at the Brockton/West Roxbury Veterans Administration Medical Center.[8]

McSherry wanted to determine if more intense, focused chaplain visits would affect total length of stay for nonsurgical patients, postoperative length of stay for surgical patients, and total dollars of hospital resources used per patient. Her team divided over seven hundred volunteer patients into eight major diagnosis categories, then randomly assigned them to three groups: those who received daily chaplain interventions from specially trained clergy; those who received a daily cheer-up humanitarian volunteer visit; and those who received no special chaplain visit beyond normal hospital care, which included a few "standard" chaplain calls.

The daily chaplain interventions were structured to meet patients' individual needs, be they certain prayers or personal discussions, as determined from the spiritual "workup" originally obtained in the structured diagnostic assessment. I must point out that this type of chaplain visit went far beyond those I knew as a young doctor, in which the patient, not the clergy member, shaped the encounter. In the "modern" chaplain-patient meeting Dr. McSherry had helped pioneer, the chaplain worked toward specific treatment goals.

John Fassett: Prayer Warrior

She chose two men with long experience in pastoral care to work with her. John Fassett, then in his mid-seventies, was senior chaplain at the Brockton/West Roxbury VA Medical Center. Former navy commander John Robert Bliss, a retired military chaplain and Episcopalian lay minister, was devoting his second career to helping modernize pastoral care at the hospital.

In more than thirty years as a chaplain at Brockton/West Roxbury, John Fassett had seen the full gamut of patients, ranging from World War II amputees suffering deep depression to young Gulf War vets terribly maimed in tank battles with the Iraqi Republican Guards. Fassett

himself was a rather crusty World War II coast guard veteran who had
survived North Atlantic convoys battling Nazi U-boats and dodging
icebergs. Although he wore his clerical "dog collar" in the hospital and
was a deeply committed Christian, John Fassett knew he often had to
employ unorthodox methods to punch through the defensive shell of
some patients to reach their spiritual core.

He was enthusiastic when Dr. McSherry described the project. "I'm
convinced the VA's chaplain service is missing the boat when it comes
to recognizing the power of prayer to improve patients' conditions," she
told Fassett and Bliss. "But we have no proof in the scientific sense."

She described the structure of her proposed study, with its control
group and rigorous double-blind framework to minimize the effects of
chance. "If you're willing to help me," she told the two chaplains, "we'll
be able to explore the power of prayer on the ward level."

Fassett and Bliss readily agreed to participate. Dr. McSherry went to
work with them, explaining the use of the innovative Spiritual Profile
Assessment.

Once the study began, John Fassett attacked his assignment with the
enthusiasm he had always brought to his profession. He contacted the
patients in his group on the day they were admitted to the hospital, often lingering outside their rooms to enter as soon as the residents had
completed the standard medical admissions chart. "Look," Fassett always said, handing over the clipboard with the questionnaire. "You
don't have to do this. But we'd like you to help your country even more
than you already have."

That approach worked well with a variety of Protestant, Catholic,
and Jewish veterans admitted for open-heart surgery.

Once having established initial rapport, Fassett carefully studied the
information in the SPA, searching for individual traits he might work
on to cement a spiritual bond.

In the profile of one Korean War veteran in his mid-sixties, for example, Fassett read that the man was practically paralyzed with death
anxiety before his heart-bypass surgery. Fassett realized the veteran
probably suffered unresolved combat stress dating back more than forty
years and was now focusing those decades of anxiety on his heart opera-

tion. Although the surgery went well, Fassett found the veteran looking wan and dejected as he shuffled down the corridor, listlessly push-
ing his IV trolley. *He's still wound up tight with fear,* Fassett realized.
Then he saw the man begin to tremble violently, the color draining
from his cheeks, his lips taking on a sickly blue tinge. He was going into
heart arrhythmia, probably as much from anxiety as from standard
postsurgical complications.

Fassett led the man to his bed and spoke in a soothing tone. "You *are*
going to be all right," he assured the rigid figure lying before him. "Just
think of yourself stretched out on a picnic blanket in a nice park on a
sunny June day. Your toes aren't shaking; neither are your feet. Your
whole body is beginning to relax. . . ." Indeed, the man's rigid frame
sagged into the sheets and his tense jaw muscles loosened.

"It's Sunday, time to say a little prayer," Fassett continued. "Our Father, who art in heaven. . . ." Before Fassett had finished the Lord's
Prayer, the man was sleeping peacefully.

Later, in the study, Fassett encountered a veteran he recalls as "a
hard nut to crack." The man's SPA revealed he had no religious affiliation, had not attended services since childhood, and was depressed
about his serious heart condition, which required a triple coronary
artery bypass. He was also bitter about his family, Fassett noted: The
man's children, according to the SPA, had "gone wild," slipping into a
morass of drugs, petty crime, and messy divorces that left behind an
embittered throng of former in-laws who did all they could to prevent
the man and his wife from visiting their grandchildren. *No wonder he's
got heart trouble,* Fassett realized.

He made sure to be in the intensive care unit when the man was
wheeled back from the operating room. Emerging from anesthesia, the
man looked up and focused slowly on Fassett's clerical collar. "Good
God," the man moaned. "Is it *that* bad?"

John smiled. "I think you're going to be okay. The doctors have
done all they can. Have you ever thought of a power higher than medicine, higher than yourself?"

"No," the man said stubbornly. "Are you asking me to pray? I won't.
You do it, that's your job."

John Fassett shook his head, showing he could be just as stubborn. "I won't pray alone, but I will make you a deal. I'm going to read the Twenty-third Psalm. It's the story of man's walk through life. *If* you like what you hear, you can say 'Amen' afterward."

The man nodded, but didn't speak.

" 'The Lord is my shepherd; I shall not want. . . .' "

By the time Fassett completed the psalm, the man's eyes were filled with tears. "God *damn*," he muttered. "I never said 'Amen' before, but I'll say it now. Amen."

Chaplain John Fassett had succeeded in piercing this lonely, bitter man's depressive shell and reaching his vulnerable core of spirituality.

The McSherry Study's Findings

When the study was completed in 1992, McSherry's team found that all the patients who received Fassett and Bliss's specialized daily chaplain visits had consistently shorter hospital stays and had used fewer hospital resources than their counterparts who were not visited daily by the trained chaplains.

Major open-heart surgery patients who received the special daily chaplain visits averaged an impressive two-day decrease in length of stay, compared with their counterparts who did not receive the specialized pastoral intervention. And the patients receiving the extra pastoral care also suffered less postsurgery depression, a finding which has great potential significance, given what we have discovered about the relationship between depression and coronary artery disease.

All told, McSherry predicted, hospitals nationwide could save as much as four thousand dollars per patient stay if they made better use of their pastoral care programs. And, she added, the cost per patient of salaried VA chaplains averaged only a hundred dollars.

"We are slowly getting out the message that pastoral care pays off," Dr. McSherry said recently. "But I have to admit this has been an uphill battle."

Unfortunately, I must agree with her. Even at a forward-looking medical center such as Duke University's, cooperation between health care professionals and chaplains has been slow in coming. For many years at my hospital, a member of the clergy had to obtain a written order from a psychiatrist to visit a patient hospitalized for depression. The rationale for this virtual fire wall between mind, body, and spirit was that pastoral counseling, which usually involved prayer, might somehow interfere with the mental health care of the patient.

But the cooperation between pastoral care people and medical professionals has improved at Duke and other leading hospitals in recent years. In fact, a survey conducted by Yankelovich Partners, and published in December 1997, of three hundred HMO executives revealed that a dramatic 94 percent were confident that prayer, meditation, and other spiritual activity such as group worship and scriptural reading could favorably augment the treatment of sick people.[9]

This belief in the healing power of faith is spreading in the health care industry. Fred Brown, the chief executive officer of the hospital consortium BJC, in St. Louis, has expanded the role and increased the budget and staff of the pastoral care program in his system. He based this decision partially on the graphic evidence of shorter hospital stays and cost saving shown in Elisabeth McSherry's research.

In many ways it's ironic that cost-conscious health care executives are rediscovering the connection between hospitals and the clergy, which reflects the traditional Judeo-Christian view of the bond between body and spirit. One of the founders of the modern hospital tradition in the West was an eleventh-century monk named Brother Gerard, who tended sick pilgrims at the church of St. John the Baptist in Jerusalem after the Crusaders conquered the Holy Land. Brother Gerard's fellow monks expanded hospital centers throughout other Christian strongholds in the Holy Land over the next two hundred years, and were the founders of the Knights Hospitaller. Their order continued to commingle medicine and religion—as well as military prowess—for several more centuries. But by the time I began to study medicine, there definitely was a barrier as impassable as any medieval castle moat between "scientific" medicine and what some of my professors dubbed the "superstition" of religion.

Brenda Peterson's Healing Ministry

One person who has seen this gap close in the past twenty years is Rev. Brenda Peterson, director of pastoral care at Methodist Hospital of Southern California, in Arcadia, east of Los Angeles. Today she juggles a demanding schedule teaching new chaplains, consulting with medical colleagues about patient care, and helping hospitalized people and their families deal with the spiritual dimensions of their illnesses.

But nineteen years ago, when Rev. Peterson began work at the hospital as a newly ordained minister, she confronted many of the obstacles that traditional medical practices had placed between clergy and the "real" health care professionals—the internists, oncologists, and surgeons who formed the elite of the hospital staff. As at Duke Hospital, chaplains at Brenda's institution needed special permission to visit the psychiatric ward.

"Then, the prevailing opinion was that religion *caused* most mental illness," Rev. Peterson now notes with an ironic chuckle. "But there have been truly radical changes, not only here, but at most major hospitals around the country," she adds. Today, at least a quarter of the patients she prays with and counsels have been admitted with psychiatric problems.

Brenda Peterson and the chaplains on her staff also form an integral part of each patient's care team, which includes hospital resident and specialized physicians, nurses, and other therapists. "Doctors and HMO executives are reading the literature about the benefits of pastoral care," she emphasizes. "For them, this is a bottom-line issue. Praying with and counseling patients makes them feel better emotionally and physically. They are ready for discharge earlier." So, the services of her pastoral care department are much in demand. "Now it's the doctors themselves who are asking us to spend time with patients," she emphasizes.

This radical change began in California about ten years ago, when laws concerning living wills and placing limits on resuscitation efforts took effect. "The medical profession had to face the issue of patient autonomy," Rev. Peterson says. To Brenda and her fellow clergy, patients' spiritual lives had always been vital; now the scientific health care professionals had to begin thinking in terms of whole-person medicine. Medical ethics assumed new prominence. It was now no longer enough to perform dexterous surgery or successfully defeat a stubborn infection; hospitals across America had to provide a "caring environment."

And the emotional warmth inherent in spiritual counseling epitomized the warmth of whole-person care. Again, the question of healing versus cure emerges. I recall when the term "quality of life" came into common usage in my profession about ten years ago. This was, perhaps, a tacit admission that modern scientific medicine, with all its technical marvels, cannot always cure, and that improving the *total* mind, body, and spirit quality of a person's life should be a major goal of the healing professions.

Brenda Peterson will never forget the time she spent with a woman in the prime of middle age who had just been diagnosed with terminal liver cancer. For three days, as her doctors ran tests to determine the extent of the cancer's spread, the woman lay rigid and stricken in her bed, gripped by absolute and fearful insomnia that would not respond to any of the sleeping medications prescribed. Exhausted and nearly delirious, the patient mumbled incoherently, near psychosis from an overload of stress hormones and a deficit of brain neurotransmitters depleted by lack of sleep and anxiety.

"Brenda," a concerned nurse called, "can you come and sit with her? We can't do anything more to help her."

Brenda Peterson brought her Bible, stroked the woman's face with a cool cloth, then began reading the comforting, ancient verses of the Psalms, just as Rachel Cowan had done with her terminally ill husband, Paul. Gradually slowing the cadence of the recitation, Brenda hoped to lull the patient into sleep. But the woman would not be soothed by scripture, as Paul Cowan had been. She remained awake, racked by deep anxiety.

Finally she rolled on her side and took both the minister's hands. "I don't know why I'm so terrified," she said with utter exhaustion. "I've always been devout and death has never really scared me. But now I feel that God has just gone away."

Brenda Peterson understood the deep spiritual void surrounding this anguished woman. Closing the Bible, she asked her casual questions about her life. Gradually, the woman spoke of her pleasant childhood, a son's marriage to a wonderful girl, the healing of an ill grandchild, the unbending support of her family.

"It seems to me that you've been blessed," Rev. Peterson commented, almost as an aside.

"Blessed?" the woman asked. Then her rigid neck and shoulders relaxed slightly. "Yes . . . I have lived a good life."

"God has been with you during all those good times," Brenda said. She glanced around the dim hospital room. "I think He's still here."

For the first time in three days, the woman smiled. "I'm beginning to feel Him around us."

She cradled her head in a crook of an arm and closed her eyes. Brenda opened the Bible and began to read again, this time from the Gospels. Within minutes, the woman was asleep.

Three days later, when all the scans and lab tests were complete, she was discharged to her home with a poor prognosis. Yet she was free of pain. She spent her last six weeks with her loved ones, sleeping well at night, and praying peacefully.

Today Brenda Peterson prays almost daily with seriously ill patients. It is normal for her to walk into the glittering tiled confines of an operating room, squeezing between hissing anesthesia and humming scanning equipment to complete a long prayer before the patient goes to sleep for surgery. She will read scripture in the eerie blue glow of CT or MRI monitors, keeping eye contact with her patients while their bodies are probed by invisible beams. Brenda has even prayed with a man who hovered at the edge of consciousness and near death during a "code blue" heart defibrillation.

"Having someone pray for you can provide great strength," she has learned during her ministry. Patients no longer feel they are powerless, caught between the invisible forces of disease on the one hand and the soulless technology of modern medicine on the other. And bringing patients' families together in prayer also provides a type of healing beyond the reach of traditional medical procedures.

In fact, reconciliations between long-estranged parents and children, or brothers and sisters, often occur when Brenda and her colleagues play the role of spiritual brokers in the hospital room. "Forgiveness and reconciliation are two of the strongest elements in spiritual healing," she has come to understand.

Patients and their families often feel an illogical, but stubborn, anger at both God and others around them for causing the illness. People might have been devout church members all their lives, only to see their retirement blighted by stroke or cancer. Why was God punishing them? Others might have long-harbored resentment that a husband's or wife's unhealthy habits—overeating, smoking, alcohol . . . the gamut of modern vices—might lie at the root of their current illness. Brothers and sisters, especially those who shared the deprivations and anxieties of the Great Depression and World War II, might have harbored festering jealous resentments for decades.

"It is essential for anger to be vented so that healing can occur," Brenda emphasizes, "and the slow process of forgiveness based on God's unlimited and unconditional love can begin."

Compared to measuring picograms of interleukin-6 per milliliter of blood, quantifying the effect of such forgiveness and reconciliation is almost impossible. Just as Dr. Elisabeth McSherry predicted almost twenty years ago, dedicated pastoral care professionals such as Rev. Brenda Peterson and her thousands of colleagues across the country play an invaluable part in the complex and evolving process of healing.

Lillian Jones's Story

But the role that the minister, priest, rabbi, or volunteer lay counselor from the patient's own congregation plays in promoting the healing of hospitalized people remains vital. Remember, spiritual counseling from clergy and congregation members literally saved Frank Kozoman's life as he lay paralyzed in the hospital following his tragic accident.

A religious visit on Christmas Day, 1996, restored the spirit of an anguished woman named Lillian Jones. Lillian, then fifty-one, had suffered lupus erythematosus for years. The autoimmune disease attacked her joints and internal organs, causing excruciating pain and disability. In extreme cases, lupus can be one of the most dangerous of the complex autoimmune disorders. But for Lillian, the overall burden of chronic pain and debilitating fatigue sapped her spirit as well as her body.

Lillian, a widow with a daughter who was working out of state, found herself alone in a hospital room at Duke University Medical Center on this chill, bright Christmas morning. Early the next day, she was scheduled for laproscopic heart surgery to repair an atrial valve damaged by lupus.

With the holiday season, many of the elective surgery beds were empty, and the ward staffs reduced. On waking early that Christmas morning, Lillian stared out the window at the empty parking lots surrounding the vast, almost industrial hospital towers. Tomorrow morning, doctors would thread tubes with tiny cutting devices into the confines of her beating heart, snipping and sewing. Tomorrow morning might be her final sunrise. *Does it really matter?* she thought listlessly, reflecting on the long struggle she'd waged against her painful disease.

"I felt almost stuck in outer space," Lillian remembers. Indeed, her emotional isolation and the spiritual void surrounding her were almost as painful as the throbbing ache in her hips, shoulders, and arms.

The nurses coming and going that morning with their Santa Claus hats and potted poinsettias tried to cheer Lillian. But she remained gripped by anguish. Then Lillian heard a bustle outside the door and Father Patrick Tuttle, a priest from Immaculate Conception Catholic Church in Durham, arrived with Lillian's close friend from church, Mary Gentile.

"We haven't forgotten you," Father Patrick said, offering Lillian a beautifully embossed Christmas card. But the young priest carried a gift far more valuable than the card in his leather satchel. With Mary assisting, Father Patrick set up his portable mass liturgical set and donned a bright vestment.

Lillian gazed at the process with mounting pleasure, mixed with awe. Raised in a devout Catholic family in New York, she'd attended parochial schools at which daily mass and Communion was a habit. During those years, she'd become accustomed to viewing the ancient liturgy at the altar as a passive, somewhat distant participant. Now this pleasant young priest had constructed an altar at the side of her hospital bed.

In many ways, Father Patrick Tuttle and Mary Gentile were mirroring the building of the symbolic Sukkoth Feast of Tabernacles booth that Paul Cowan's congregation members had constructed in his isolation room in the New York hospital. But instead of paper boughs and sheaths, they had built a symbolic cathedral.

Father Patrick read and chanted the friendly verses of the New American mass liturgy. When he reached the spiritual core of the mass, Communion, he passed the miniature chalice, draped in pressed linen, to Lillian. Swallowing the Host, Lillian was overcome with a warm, reassuring presence she had not felt for years. The cold isolation that had gripped her in these beige concrete towers beneath the thin winter Carolina sun had disappeared completely.

Following the mass, as he packed the liturgical kit, Father Patrick chuckled. "That was good wine. But if I perform more hospital masses, I'm going to become one happy priest."

Lillian stretched comfortably in bed, relishing the inner peace. "I'm ready for tomorrow," she said softly. "But the way I feel now, maybe the operation won't even be necessary."

Lillian did have her surgery. And she recovered well. Reflecting on the Christmas Day mass in that lonely hospital room, she says with deep emotion, "This was the most uplifting experience of my life."

The Future of Pastoral Care

Researchers Larry VandeCreek and Barbara Cooke are among the first to have studied the widely overlooked contribution that local ministers, priests, and rabbis make every day (and on many snowy nights) to the spiritual healing of their congregation members.[10] The researchers conclude that pastoral care of the ill is one of the most time-consuming aspects of these clergy members' hectic professional schedules. Yet the benefits in terms of improved physical health (cure) and better emotional outlook (healing) has not yet been scientifically studied on a large scale.

I certainly agree with VandeCreek and Cooke that the healing professions should investigate the economic and human benefits of this long-neglected resource.

Chapter Eleven

✳

A Disease-Prevention Model for the Twenty-first Century

Disease Prevention: The Traditional View

When I was a young medical student in the mid-1970s, my professors taught me a lot about the diagnosis and treatment of disease, but much less about its prevention among the people I would care for as a doctor. In my third year, I began making ward rounds with fellow students, joining an experienced physician to discuss the cases of hospitalized patients.

We learned to analyze the squiggles on the long paper ribbon of electrocardiogram charts to detect the telltale patterns of heart muscle damage from myocardial infarction.

But there was less information in our curriculum about the benefits of a high-fiber, low-fat diet rich in fruits and vegetables, accompanied by regular exercise, to control weight and blood pressure, which might actually help *prevent* heart disease. Looking back further to my undergraduate years at Stanford, the lack of awareness about the power of prevention in maintaining health was even more glaring: Some of my instructors, for example, smoked while they lectured our premed classes about the biology of cancer.

When Nobel Laureate chemist Linus Pauling, one of my chemistry professors at Stanford who helped create the science of molecular biology, proposed that the antioxidant properties of vitamin C might prevent many diseases, the medical establishment scoffed.

Before about 1980, conventional wisdom held that all the major advances in preventive medicine had already been made. And there was no doubt that progress had been impressive over the previous two centuries. Inoculation, modern sewage systems, and clean water supplies had eradicated such diseases as smallpox, polio, cholera, typhoid, and typhus, all of which had once haunted Europe and America. But many of my medical professors believed that little could be done to stop the inevitable onset of what the World Health Organization has called the "diseases of affluence": diabetes, cancer, and cardiovascular disease.

Disease Prevention: The Second Revolution

Since then, of course, there has been a second prevention revolution in medicine. On the eve of the new millennium, bright high school seniors can probably tell you more than you really want to know about antioxidants and cancer prevention. And smokers in America are practically social outcasts.

But when I was a young family practitioner visiting patients like the Clevengers in rural Missouri, this preventive medicine revolution was just beginning. There was still a big gap between what doctors felt intuitively about the relationship between diet (or smoking) and disease and a solid base of scientific research findings that proved these assumptions.

That gap no longer exists. Thousands of research projects and numerous multidecade investigations such as the Framington (Massachusetts) Heart Study and the National Institutes of Health Establishment of Populations for Epidemiologic Studies of the Elderly have provided persuasive evidence of links between diet, exercise, obesity, blood pressure, and cardiovascular disease. Although the causative connection between lifestyle factors and many forms of cancer does not have a firm grounding in research, many health-conscious people, especially in my generation, firmly believe that the type and quantity of food they eat, their level of fitness, and their consumption of vitamin and mineral supplements offer them some protection from cancer and heart problems.

And the chances are your local HMO is focused on preventive medicine—including regular periodic disease screening, weight and blood pressure control, encouragement of exercise, and cessation of smoking—in a way few would have predicted when I began medical school. One reason for this shift toward avoiding or delaying the onset of chronic illness is clear: It is easier to prevent a disease than to treat it. It is also cheaper, a major consideration in today's health care industry.

The U.S. Public Health Service formalized preventive health as a national goal when in 1991 it published *Healthy People 2000: National Health Promotion and Disease Prevention*. This massive work drew upon the exhaustive research that had slowly accrued over previous decades. I believe the following paragraph from the introduction is worth repeating to demonstrate the dramatic shift toward prevention that has occurred in medicine:

> We have learned that a fuller measure of health, a better quality of life, is within our personal grasp. If tobacco use in this country stopped entirely today, an estimated 390,000 fewer Americans would die before their time each year. If all Americans reduced their consumption of foods high in fat to well below current levels and engaged in physical activity no more strenuous than sustained walking for 30 minutes a day, additional results of similar magnitude could be expected. If alcohol were never carelessly used in our society, about 100,000 fewer people would die from unnecessary illness and injury. Together, deaths from these causes comprise a sizable share of the 2.1 million deaths that occur annually and are examples of the impact of personal lifestyle choices on the health destiny of individual Americans and the future of the Nation.[1]

Religion and Disease Prevention

Every time I read this passage, I'm tempted to scribble in the margin of the book: "If every American became religiously or spiritually active and followed the healthy tenets of his or her faith, our nation might achieve *most* of these laudable goals." Certainly I hope that if *Healthy*

People is ever revised, the authors will highlight the possible disease prevention aspects of religious faith.

But, for the moment, clinicians on the front line of patient care are only slowly learning to incorporate the potential of faith's healing power into the preventive medicine they practice each day. This cautious approach to the melding of religion and medicine has long been justified because there simply has not been enough scientific evidence that religious faith and involvement produce tangible benefits to physical and emotional health. That situation is beginning to change.

In 1993, the privately funded National Institute for Healthcare Research in Rockville, Maryland, assembled hundreds of studies on the health benefits of religious faith and activity into a research guide called "The Faith Factor."

The NIHR found that 77 percent of studies on the health benefits of religion demonstrate a positive effect, including in the areas of drug and alcohol abuse, emotional illness, chronic pain, cardiovascular disease, and general health. Perhaps most interesting, religious faith was shown to increase people's overall survival rates.

Since this research guide was released six years ago, I'm pleased to report, the healing power of faith has gained increasing respect in the medical establishment. In 1997, for example, Jeffrey Levin, Ph.D., and David Larson, M.D., both of the NIHR, and Christina Puchalski, M.D., of George Washington School of Medicine, wrote an insightful summary of American medicine's growing acceptance of the faith-health connection in one of the world's most prestigious, peer-reviewed scientific publications, the *Journal of the American Medical Association*.[2]

They cited the steadily accumulating research evidence that religious involvement is a "protective factor" that can be quantified like other health variables such as diet, exercise, smoking, or alcohol use. They also noted that researchers have begun addressing the "why" question by trying to identify emotional and biological pathways "through which religious or spiritual practice may promote health or prevent disease."

Research on the broad health aspects of religious faith, the authors noted, "has increased the validity of religion and spirituality as topics for still further medical research." This has led the National Institutes of Health, the federal government's leading biomedical research organization, to fund a number of important studies in this area.

If the medical establishment's recognition of religion's value has not come full circle from the days of the Knights Hospitaller, it's certainly moved forward since I earned my M.D. For example, Harvard Medical School, Dr. Herbert Benson's Mind-Body Medical Institute, and Beth Israel Deaconess Medical Center in Boston now present regular seminars—called "Spirituality & Healing"—that are attended by leading health professionals from many disciplines. One major thrust of these conferences is the wellness-enhancing or preventive benefit of religious faith and involvement.

The importance of the relationship between spirituality and health continues to spread among our leading medical educators. Last year, the John Templeton Foundation awarded its latest round of grants to eight of America's top medical schools to develop courses that explore the connection between health and religion in patient care. These institutions include the schools of medicine at Brown, Georgetown, and Morehouse Universities, plus the University of Chicago, hardly obscure "Bible colleges." Dr. Aaron E. Glatt, a professor at Albert Einstein College of Medicine, who helped develop a course entitled, "Faith and Medicine: An Oxymoron?" which received a Templeton curriculum grant in 1995, is enthusiastic about the new interest in exploring the healing power of faith that the medical establishment is beginning to show. "There's another world—the world of the human spirit—that medical students don't learn about in school but will encounter in their practices," Dr. Glatt emphasizes. "As physicians, they won't always have the answers to spiritual-medical issues, but they should learn to ask the questions and point their patients in the direction for help."

Another positive aspect of this new interest in the health-faith link is the growing recognition that the once-nebulous mind-body connection is a critical factor in the whole-person medicine that many clinicians now try to practice. The influence of both positive and negative emotional states—optimism and well-being as well as distress and depression—over the body has now been well documented.[3] In fact, much of the evidence for the healing power of religious faith lies in this connection.

As I described in Chapter One, in 1996 the American Association for the Advancement of Science allowed me and several colleagues who had long been struggling in the research wilderness to present papers at a symposium titled, "Religious Factors that Influence Disease States."

The New Prevention Model

My principal contribution was discussing research on the relationship between religion, depression, and physical health that stemmed from a multiyear study of older people I led with my Duke University research team.[4] We investigated this relationship in the random sample of four thousand people over age sixty-five participating in the Duke University site of the national EPESE study.

Once more, our major findings were revealing:

• Overall level of religious activity was positively related to good physical health and negatively related to depressive symptoms. In other words, religiously active people seemed to enjoy better emotional health and to have fewer physical health problems than the less religious.
• Splitting religion into public and private activity, we found that frequent church attenders, in particular, were physically healthier and less depressed than infrequent attenders (those who were attending less than once per week).

This research project, more than any other study I've worked on, led me toward the creation of the "Prevention Model for Religion's Effects on Physical Health" diagram. In my research team's discussion of the findings, we noted:

The positive relationship between church attendance and good physical health, however, is also consistent with a protective effect. Active involvement in a religious community may protect against physical health problems in a number of ways. First, frequent church attendance may keep older persons mobile and active, which then helps to prevent further functional decline. Second, it may increase one's social network, which then enhances monitoring for health problems (increasing disease detection and treatment) and perhaps compliance with treatment. Third, it may reduce high-risk behaviors (smoking, alcohol use, etc.) associated with health problems. Fourth, it may help reduce emotional distress, which has been linked with various psychosomatic diseases.

Our work was well received at the meeting, but many of the scientists attending wanted to explore the actual biological pathways through which active religious faith might prevent disease and promote wellness.

It was to provide medical professionals this understanding—and also to offer average people a better understanding of religion's health-promotion qualities—that I began working on the "Prevention Model for Religion's Effects on Health."

The links shown in this model are continually being confirmed by rigorous studies now being published in medical journals.

This diagram (see page 262) is a blueprint for researchers trying to understand the complex relationships and processes involved in religion's effects on human health. Creating a visual representation of the ways in which religious faith interacts with people's lives, and through this interaction influences their health, has allowed me and my colleagues to better grasp the major elements involved in the relationship between religious faith and health.

You can think of the model as a schematic summary of the material presented in this book. But keep in mind that this diagram is an abstraction of a vastly more complex set of real-world interactions. In the model, the lines of causation are straight; in the intricate web of events, habits, beliefs, love, and antipathy that make up people's actual lives, many of these connections are more subtle and harder to disentangle.

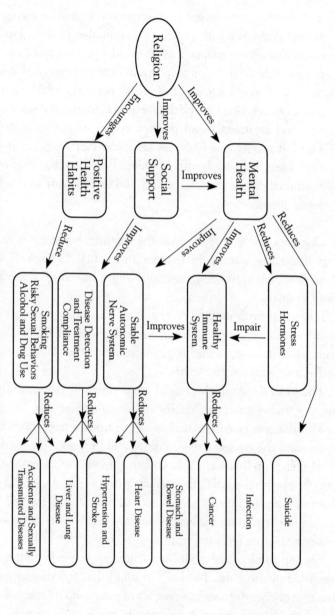

Adapted from *Is Religion Good for Your Health?* (Binghamton, NY: Haworth Press, 1997). Used with permission.

In the model, "Religion" is defined as a combination of both a strong personal belief and involvement with that faith, such as private religious activities (prayer, scripture reading), use of religion to help cope with stress, frequency of attendance at services, and participation in congregational activities.

The arrows represent connections among the major elements of the health-religion relationship: religious faith and practice; social support from friends and family; mental (emotional) health; the immune system; and the autonomic nervous system. The other arrows indicate direct pathways from these elements to several major categories of physical health and disease.

For example, let's briefly examine the visual representation of cause and effect in the model. How does religion affect mental health and how does this influence physical health? Research shows that faith improves mental health by helping people cope well with life stressors, which reduces overproduction of stress hormones. Lower levels of stress hormones, in turn, will result in less impairment of the immune system and thereby reduce the risk of certain infections or cancers. The role of religion in bolstering social support can also help people cope with stress, alleviate anxiety, and prevent depression. This further helps reduce levels of the stress hormones and prevents the autonomic nervous system from becoming hyperactive, thus lowering blood pressure and decreasing risk of heart disease and stroke.

So, as the model indicates, the connection between emotional and physical health is one of the *key* elements in explaining the physiological pathways involved in religion's health-enhancing powers.

A Scientific Model

I want to emphasize that I have not included divine intervention in my disease prevention model. I am concerned here only with what can be examined and tested by the scientific method. I happen to be a person of faith, but I am also a scientist and a physician. This model is rooted firmly in the known psychological, social, and physiological laws of science.

Religious faith and practice may positively influence people's health both indirectly and directly.

Indirect Health Benefits of Religion: The Bonds of Faith

As we've seen throughout the book, belonging to an emotionally supportive spiritual community gives people a sense of life satisfaction and transcendental purpose. Involved in religion's indirect effect on health are the enriching support of a person's network of concerned friends, the strengthening of marriage and family bonds, and the mitigation of life stress, anxiety, and depression.

A major pathway derives from the social support people receive through belonging to a faith community. "Social Support" in the model refers to the strong personal bonds that develop among members of a congregation. You'll recall that in one of my first research projects in the Midwest I found that many older people drew most of their closest friends from their church congregations. And you'll also remember that it was a chance encounter with a religious young man at a Friday Sabbath service that turned Dan's life around and ultimately helped save his marriage and preserve his family. The dry scientific term "social support" cannot adequately describe the deep emotional bonds that developed between Frank Kozoman and the people in his congregation after his accident left him paralyzed. Without their love and concern, he would not have survived. If you think of similar stories, repeated over and over again, you'll begin to see the human face that this element of the model represents.

The positive effect of close friendships within a congregation on emotional health cannot be overstated. Shelly Cole's long battle with suicidal depression, which was never controlled by conventional medication or psychotherapy, only ended when her sister brought her into the warm bonds of a concerned congregation. In a similar manner, Chris Benfield's odyssey of adolescent self-destruction was not resolved until he found a spiritual home provided by the youth outreach ministry of a charismatic Christian church. Deep religious faith and the strong support of Deliverance Evangelistic Church's Drug Task Force empowered Rick to break the bonds of heroin addiction and to go on to a productive life.

Religious faith and involvement improve well-being by decreasing the effects of stress, anxiety, and depression.

For many people not protected by faith, the stresses of hectic daily life and especially troubling events such as divorce or bereavement provoke a slide into depression. As we've seen, this in turn causes overproduction of the stress hormones—cortisol, epinephrine, and norepinephrine—which are released by the adrenal glands. These stress hormones overstimulate the autonomic nervous system, increasing blood pressure and heart and respiration rates, and often leading to cardiovascular disease.

The cascade of the stress hormone cortisol unleashed by chronic depression can also affect the immune system. In turn, a weakened immune system leaves a person vulnerable to infections, several forms of cancer, and the buildup of atherosclerotic plaque in the blood vessels that can lead to heart attacks and stroke.[5]

In January 1998, Bruce S. McEwen, Ph.D., a nationally recognized physiology expert, read an insightful paper on the effects of chronic stress on the body at a medical seminar sponsored by Beth Israel Deaconess Medical Center in Boston. Dr. McEwen summarized the latest findings in this field of study, which strongly suggest there is a powerful link between unmitigated stress and physical problems due to a weakened immune system and increased vulnerability to cardiovascular disease.[6]

Chronic stress and anxiety, as well as more significant depression, cause overactivity in our most basic neurological network—the autonomic nervous system, which controls the unconscious functions of breathing, blood circulation, digestion, and intestinal activity. If long-term emotional distress hyperactivates the autonomic nervous system, people are at greater risk of digestive problems, including irritable bowel syndrome, which can be quite serious.

But extended autonomic nervous system overactivity also has a dramatic impact on cardiovascular health, and is clearly associated with increased risk of high blood pressure and heart disease.[7]

                                    ✳

Summarizing this aspect of faith's preventive power, research has shown:

- Religious people are shielded from depression and recover faster if afflicted than their less religious counterparts.
- Religion is often a significant factor in preventing suicide, which is now threatening adolescents as well as adults.
- People who both attend church frequently and for whom faith is an important part of their lives have consistently lower blood pressure than the less religiously active.
- There is a link between level of religious involvement and heart disease: In general, the deeper a person's faith, as measured by degree of orthodoxy or frequency of attendance at religious services, the lower the risk of heart attack.

So, the *indirect* effects of religion in bolstering social support and improving emotional health have been well established by scientific research and form an important part of the framework in the "Prevention Model."

The Direct Benefits of Religion: Respect for the Body

The *direct* preventive health effects of religion follow two pathways.

First, research shows that religious people with a strong social support network often have their diseases diagnosed earlier, become actively involved in their treatment, and follow their caregivers' instructions (i.e., take their medicines correctly, follow a restricted diet) more closely than less religious people. This may be because a wide range of denominations within the Judeo-Christian heritage tend to pay heightened respect to the human body as the pinnacle of God's creation. The Book of Genesis, for example, teaches that Adam and Eve were created "in the image of God . . . male and female." For many Christians, the human body is a "temple" of the Holy Spirit. Therefore it's not surprising that research has shown that religiously involved people are more compliant with medical treatment and more likely to follow the guidance and advice of their caregivers.

We've also seen that religious people have stronger marriages, in which love and trust build the type of lifelong intimacy that transcends the self-absorption that has marked many relationships. Husbands and wives in religious marriages are often deeply concerned about each other and are likely to encourage their spouses toward disease screening and early treatment for health problems.

This degree of loving concern also often exists among members of a congregational "family," who encourage each other to maintain good health. And the faith community of a church or synagogue has proven to be an excellent setting for health promotion and wellness education programs.

In the late 1980s, the Pawtucket Heart Health Program in Rhode Island studied the impact of community-wide health education and found that large groups of adults could be motivated to reduce their risk of serious cardiovascular disease significantly by educating fellow congregation members about the dangers of smoking, high blood pressure, elevated cholesterol, obesity, and lack of exercise. Researchers found that church-based programs using volunteers to manage these education efforts was one of the most efficient means of spreading the word about cardiovascular health.[8]

Today, such health education programs exist in religious congregations across the country. Church-based "wellness centers," which began slowly with the second preventive medicine revolution in the 1980s, are steadily spreading. One of the first regional networks of such centers was New England's computerized Church Information System, which linked 8,200 churches and synagogues for the sharing of resource information and curricula about health promotion. In the South, Dr. James Alley, former director of Georgia's Public Health Department, helped lead the development of health-promotion outreach efforts in both black and white churches. And you'll also recall that religiously based weight-control programs are steadily spreading across the country.

Some congregations rely on volunteer health care professionals to help with annual cholesterol and diabetes screenings, nutrition classes, and education on risk factors of other diseases. In many congregations, as we have noted, the parish nurse program has taken firm root. All of this wellness outreach shares the common bond of fraternal love among congregation members.

Loving Concern: Dr. Iris Keys

A good example of this mingling of fellowship and professional concern for preventive health is found in the life and work of Baltimore physician Iris Keys. A thoughtful and serene African-American woman in her fifties, Dr. Keys did not enter medical school until she was forty years old. Today she has a busy practice at the University of Maryland Medical Center in downtown Baltimore, with many of her patients older African-American women.

Dr. Keys has a definite advantage in establishing empathy with her patients and helping them to develop healthier lifestyle habits to combat serious conditions such as diabetes and cardiovascular disease. She is an ordained minister in the AME Church, the denomination to which many of these people belong. Her patients trust Iris Keys not only for her medical expertise, but also for her spirituality.

When Iris Keys is invited to a church, she says, "I preach the Gospel and good health."

Indeed, Iris Keys spends much of her free time discussing cardiovascular health with Baltimore's black church congregations. An expert in blood pressure control, she has chosen as her mission educating her "brothers and sisters in Christ" about the risks and avoidance of hypertension that plagues the African-American community. "I can mix sound medical advice with 'church talk,' " Dr. Keys adds.

Her work follows the pioneering Baltimore Church High Blood Pressure Program research project, which began in the mid-1980s. The study found that Baltimore churches were an excellent setting to educate black women on weight loss and blood pressure control through exercise and medication. Many of the women participating in the two-year study enjoyed significant reductions in both weight and blood pressure, based on changes in their diet, exercise level, and compliance with medication, all grounded in the church-based health education project.[9]

I believe that Dr. Keys's personal and professional dedication is an excellent example of the "Prevention Model" in action.

Direct Benefits of Religion: A Healthy Lifestyle

The second health-enhancing direct effect of religious faith is the avoidance of unhealthy habits.

For example, healthier lifestyles among the religiously involved lead to lower rates of pulmonary disease such as emphysema and lung cancer (consequences of smoking), lower levels of liver disease such as cirrhosis (stemming from alcohol abuse), and significantly lower levels of other substance abuse than exist among the general population.[10] Dr. Kenneth Kendler of Virginia Commonwealth University found during his groundbreaking research on twins: "Religiosity may be one of the more important familial-environmental factors that affect the risk of substance abuse and dependence."[11]

It's worth noting that our research at Duke has shown that, even among men of the World War II generation born and raised in the heart of North Carolina's tobacco country, the religiously devout were significantly less likely to have ever smoked. If we consider the abstemious ways of conservative Protestants in general—avoiding both alcohol and smoking, and exerting strong pressure against sexual promiscuity—it becomes clear that this type of faith milieu has overall health-promotion qualities.

And rates of sexually transmitted disease are lower among the religious than among their nonreligious peers. For example, during the sexual revolution of the 1960s, very little was said about one of the most severe sexually transmitted diseases, cervical cancer, which is carried by the human papilloma virus. Avoiding unprotected sexual intercourse with multiple partners decreases risk of the disease. In the 1970s, researchers in Utah found significantly lower rates of cervical cancer in Mormon women compared with both their non-Mormon peers in the state and the national average.[12] This lower incidence might well stem from the more constrained sexual practices of Mormons in Utah, where church doctrine has long set prevailing cultural patterns.

A Life of Healthy Faith: Steve and Martha Bollinger's Story

The long and successful marriage of Steve and Martha Bollinger is another living example of faith's healing power, as diagrammed in the "Prevention Model."

Steve and Martha, both fifty-one, met as children in Sunday school at the United Methodist Church in the small town of Jackson, Missouri. In many ways, their life together has been as much a spiritual odyssey as a human partnership of love and devotion.

They both came from hardworking families. Martha's father was a machinist, her mother an office worker. After working in local factories, Steve's father saved enough to buy a small general store at a dusty crossroads outside of town.

"Even before we went to high school," Steve remembers, "I had made a commitment to devote my life in service to the Lord in whatever way He showed me."

"Steve's faith," Martha notes four decades after they met, "was one of the reasons I fell in love with him."

In high school, neither of them really doubted who they would marry. Steve earned a teaching degree at the local college, while Martha became a hairdresser. They married when Steve received his bachelor's degree in 1968. Rather than teach, however, Steve enrolled in dental school, and Martha worked long hours to support them. Their first son, Todd, was born between Steve's second and third years of dental school.

Steve recalls those years happily. "We were really very busy, but we always recognized we were partners."

"We learned how to trust God," Martha adds.

The couple spent two years at Fort Dix, New Jersey, where their second son, Matthew, was born, and Steve completed his military obligation as an army dentist. Then they came home to Missouri in the mid-1970s and Steve buckled down to the hard work and financial strain of establishing a dental practice.

Steve and Martha had learned early in life to use prayer, Bible study, and church to ease the inevitable stress of life. And the stress level was steadily increasing across the country. Today, for example, there is little doubt that life stress has become a serious concern for many families. A colleague at Duke University Medical Center, Linda J. Luecken, M.D., investigated the levels of stress hormones in working women and found that working mothers reported more stress and less sense of control than women without children living at home.[13] Dr. Luecken noted that such chronic stress might contribute to illness among these women because the stress hormones, especially cortisol, affected their immune systems.

But the Bollingers felt strongly that God had always played an active role in their lives. So their daily stress levels rarely became severe, even though Steve was struggling to build his practice.

By 1980, Steve had an active practice and the couple's financial picture looked bright. In many ways their future was predictable: increasingly large homes, memberships in the local country club and community organizations that marked acceptance into the upper stratum of American small-town life, a few indulgences such as a luxury car, perhaps a Caribbean cruise. After all, they had worked for years to earn this secure niche.

But Steve had never forgotten his childhood commitment to religious service. One evening after dinner was over and their little boys had gone to bed, Steve and Martha spoke quietly about the future. "I guess I'm just not satisfied without serving the Lord," Steve said. Through church friends, they'd learned that a growing campus mission in North Carolina needed lay ministers. "I think this is the direction God wants us to go," Steve told Martha.

"Let's pray about it," she said. The couple bowed their heads and joined in prayer, as they had throughout their life together.

By the end of the evening, it was clear to both of them that leaving the world of conventional success to embark on this ministry was indeed the direction God intended their life to follow.

Within weeks, the Bollingers had sold most of their possessions and Steve's hard-won dental practice. Early one morning, they left the familiar confines of Jackson, and their overloaded car headed across the Mississippi River into the hot summer sun rising over Tennessee. "This is a real step of faith," Steve told Martha.

She smiled, confident that they were following God's plan.

For many Baby Boom couples, the divorce epidemic of the 1980s was taking its toll. Columnists and popular psychologists lamented the malaise-amidst-affluence that seemed to be spreading among Baby Boomers. Stress of work pressure and personal dissatisfaction had become palpable across the country. Alcohol abuse was rampant in the suburbs. The cocaine plague had spread from urban ghettos to country-club locker rooms. But their deep religious faith and commitment shielded Steve and Martha from these problems.

Over the next seventeen years, the Bollingers worked closely together. Steve helped establish a campus ministry at the University of North Carolina and later became a teacher at a private Christian school. Martha was a stay-at-home mother and active in their church. The couple spent more than ten years living in a rental home, a definite step down from their financial security in Missouri. "But we taught our boys that there were other kinds of success in life than making a lot of money," Martha notes.

Indeed, Todd and Matthew Bollinger were raised in a happy, secure family.

At no point during these lean years did either Steve or Martha feel tempted to relieve the unavoidable stress of life through alcohol, drugs, or sexual infidelity.

In 1996, Steve's annual physical exam revealed that his blood cholesterol was rising. Even though Martha had always tried to provide the family a healthy diet, she now concentrated on eliminating much of the fat from their meals and substituting fruits and vegetables. They both fought incipient middle-age bulging by finding time in the week for exercise walking.

The Bollingers had watched with deep pride as their sons grew into adulthood and graduated from college. Through hard work and saving,

Steve and Martha had managed to buy their own suburban home. It seemed that God had indeed blessed their lives.

Then, on a hot Friday afternoon in May 1997, Martha had a mammogram as part of her annual physical. The next week, her doctor called, noting that there had been a "small spot" on her X-ray plate. He referred her to surgeon Dr. James Wilson.

"It may be nothing to worry about," Dr. Wilson advised, pointing to the chalky shadow on the plate, "but I'd like to do a biopsy."

Martha gripped Steve's hand tightly as she gazed at the lighted image. Her mouth felt dry, her hands clammy. This was every woman's nightmare.

That evening at home, Steve and Martha prayed together as they had for years, and she felt her anxiety begin to lift. "Lord," she said, head bowed in prayer, "we trust You as we always have."

The next Saturday Steve and Martha were home when Dr. Wilson called to announce sadly that the biopsy had tested positive for cancer. Martha slumped hard into a chair, her eyes clouded with tears. "Come on over to my office and let's talk about this," Dr. Wilson suggested.

Martha sat rooted in the chair, feeling the cold dread spreading through her.

Then her abiding faith returned. She and Steve said a brief prayer and drove to the doctor's office. They decided he would perform a lumpectomy in two weeks. During the interim, Martha was embraced by the loving concern of the members of her congregation. One of her church friends, Genie Lewis, whose long struggle with multiple sclerosis we described earlier, was especially comforting. "Everyone is praying hard for you," Genie reassured her.

Just after sunrise on the third Friday in May, Martha lay on a gurney, prepped for surgery, when Dr. Wilson greeted her on his way to the scrub room. Martha gripped his arm. "I just want to know one thing. Have you prayed today?"

Dr. Wilson smiled. "I pray every day."

Martha felt warm comfort. Her whole life had been in the Lord's hands. And it still was.

During the surgery, Dr. Wilson discovered that the tumor, although still localized, was larger than the mammogram image had suggested. Following Martha's request, he performed a simple mastectomy rather than the less invasive lumpectomy.

The next week, the driveway of the Bollingers' home was often crowded with the cars of church members. Women from Martha's prayer group and her women's ministry visited daily. As Martha recovered over the coming weeks, the people from church brought meals, did housework, and spent time praying with her.

"I can't imagine how people can go through something this frightening without faith," Martha says with deep feeling.

I have never heard a more heartfelt description of successful religious coping than those words. As we've seen, depression is one of the most dangerous sequelae of breast cancer. And depression, in turn, can impair the body's ability to *contain* the cancer. But Martha's deep faith has shielded her.

Although Dr. Wilson had assured Martha that all of the cancerous tissue had been excised, there were moments when she felt her fear rising again. At those times, she found great solace in praying, softly singing hymns, and reading the Bible. "Keep your eyes on the Lord," she reminded herself. The stressful fear dissolved.

You might ask why I've included Martha's story in this discussion of prevention. Doesn't the fact that she developed breast cancer suggest that the Bollingers' faith and healthy lifestyle actually *failed* to protect Martha? Not really. Biomedical science still does not understand all the risk factors for breast cancer, beyond a certain percentage of cases that can be attributed to genetic risk. We'll never know what caused Martha's tumor.

But her faith had always provided her an emotionally healthy level of self-esteem; she had believed since childhood that God was directly involved in her life. This led to a respect for her physical body as divinely created, which in turn had engendered a healthy lifestyle, including regular medical exams and disease screening. It was probably this adherence to annual mammogram guidelines that saved Martha's life, as it allowed her doctor to detect the tumor when it was still localized.

A year after her surgery, Martha Bollinger is completely recovered and again actively involved with her women's ministry.

Steve helped the church in developing a youth outreach program at a low-income housing project where many single mothers live. Over the last four years, he and his church volunteers have expanded a summer remedial reading program in a vacant apartment into a permanent tutoring center run by a full-time teacher. The children have a safe and wholesome place to study and do homework every day after school.

Although volunteering at the center during his summer vacation from teaching takes hours each week, Steve remains enthusiastic. This summer, he will begin tutoring the bright and active children in science, using a large aquarium donated by church members as his principal tool in explaining the mysteries of biology.

He finds deep satisfaction in watching the children—whom many of his more conventionally successful peers in the affluent suburbs, and on many university campuses, might consider predestined to a life of poverty—beam with sudden understanding as they watch frog eggs grow into tadpoles. Echoing Ruby Clevenger, he's optimistic about their futures. "They're God's children like the rest of us."

Steve is especially proud that some of his young students and their families have begun attending the Bollingers' church. "My goal has always been to lead others to the Lord."

Looking back on their long marriage, Martha admits that she sometimes wonders what their lives would have been like had they not left Missouri. "But I have no regrets," she says sincerely. "Faith, health, and family are more important than material wealth."

In this regard, the Bollingers share the life satisfaction and sense of optimism enjoyed by so many of the religious people we have met in this book. As a physician and medical researcher, I find Steve and Martha's story a splendid example of how the prevention model can work in real life.

Chapter Twelve

✳

Helping Yourself and Your Loved Ones Benefit from the Power of Faith

The people we've encountered in this book have spanned the country and most of the twentieth century.

They have ranged from Walter Grounds, saying his Lord's prayer as he hacked coal from an unlicensed mine in some forgotten Appalachian hollow, to Rev. Brenda Peterson, reading the words of Jesus ("I will; be thou clean . . .") in the Gospel of Matthew to a cancer patient lying beneath a radiation gun in the Los Angeles suburbs.

We've met people like Ruby and Bill Clevenger and their adopted daughter, Cindy, in the rural Midwest, who some would call poor, but who enjoy a rich abundance of faith. We have seen Monty Cox and Rick, one a white man in a small southern town, one an African-American in an inner city, both former slaves to alcohol or drugs, condemned to addiction and premature death, both now freed through their faith. We have shared a long life of faith with Louise Hudson that has taken her from rural poverty to continued dedicated service to those less fortunate than herself. We have met Chris Benfield, a tormented adolescent entranced by alcohol and the suicidal "death metal" that had lured friends toward self-destruction, but saved through finding the courage to take refuge in a power infinitely stronger than himself.

What do these disparate people have in common? They all have felt the healing power of faith. By that I mean these men and women have mobilized their spiritual lives to help overcome the hardships of physical and emotional illness, or in some cases to prevent disease, and in general have used faith to improve their quality of life and well-being.

With their successful exercise of faith in mind, and with years of practice as a physician working among people who have also been so generously blessed, I would like to now share some of what they have taught me. To accomplish this, I'd like to offer some practical suggestions to help enhance the health benefits of religion, first to people who already enjoy an active spiritual life, and secondly to those who do not have religious faith.

As you read these suggestions, keep in mind the firm foundation of evidence to support this advice that has emerged from hundreds of research studies, many of which we have discussed in detail in this book. Remember, however, that I am *not* offering spiritual counseling here, but rather trying to provide advice to enhance the health benefits of faith, based on this scientific research.

If You Already Are Religious

1. Consider attending religious services more frequently, and becoming more involved in the spiritual community of your church or synagogue. You can become an usher, a lay reader, a Sunday school teacher, a volunteer janitor or nursery worker. You can help organize potluck dinners or garage sales.

   On the spiritual side, you can join a prayer chain group, as Peggy La Vigne did. Or you can simply make an effort to reach out spiritually to people in need, as Paul Burns has done so often since his wife was stricken with Alzheimer's disease.

   One tangible benefit of all these efforts is that they help put your own worries into perspective. Remember, level of religious faith and what we call "religious giving" have consistently been associated with better emotional health.

   Another concrete advantage derived from this increased involvement with your congregation is the improved and ongoing social support you'll receive.

2. Identify your own special talents—perhaps musical, teaching, or vocational skills—and use them to help out less fortunate people in your church and local community. Try volunteering

a couple of hours per week. Become a hospital or nursing home
visitor; provide respite for someone who is homebound caring
for a sick loved one. Maybe just baby-sit children so that parents can have a night out.

Like Louise Hudson, almost ninety, who finds time to work
at a church mission, you might want to share the wisdom of
your long life of faith with young women trying to face the
world as single mothers. Or you might bring your congregation
together to join in a larger volunteer outreach program as
Steve Bollinger did.

Again, stepping outside yourself has been shown to improve
outlook, relieve anxiety, and increase one's sense of well-being.

3. Attend a prayer or scripture study group once a week. Praying
with others—as Martha Bollinger and Peggy LaVigne do during both regular service and Bible study—increases the emotional satisfaction of prayer. Keep in mind that the research
we've discussed has generally shown that *regular* prayer, scriptural reading, or study seem to provide the most health benefits.

Scripture is the foundation of all the world's monotheistic
religions. Studying scripture brings you closer to your faith. But
there is another advantage to becoming active in a study
group, especially if you are introverted and feel socially isolated: You may well gain a sense of confidence from this experience you would have trouble finding in the secular world.

4. Get up thirty minutes earlier each morning, and spend that
time in prayer; both petitionary prayer (praying to God for
something) and meditative prayer (calming your thoughts and
listening for God to answer) have been shown to enhance
health. Consider the value that Khalita Jones gains from such
spiritual discipline.

5. Take a few minutes each day, other than at mealtimes, to pray
with your spouse and children. Use this calm occasion to ask
them about conflicts in their lives and try to lift their spirits
through prayer. This is an excellent way to "disarm" anxiety
before it can snowball into depression.

✳

Family prayer also provides an excellent opportunity to express forgiveness. Remember, small unresolved emotional hurts can accumulate into larger "issues," but a simple request for and granting of forgiveness within a prayerful setting can be very healing. It's worth noting that forgiveness (atonement) plays a major part in the Judeo-Christian tradition, and that Greek Orthodox Christians still practice an annual Lenten ritual of mutual family forgiveness.

6. Make the effort to discuss religious topics with your friends and family. All the newsmagazines and major newspapers now regularly feature religious stories—a clear sign the Baby Boom generation is becoming more spiritual. But don't argue about these topics. Instead, try to listen to each other and learn; share your spiritual experiences.

As you do so, remember the healing that Chris Benfield gained when he met the young religious people on the California campus, who were so much more tolerant than the rigidly sanctimonious people he had encountered at his home church.

7. Take a few minutes out of each busy day to read religious scriptures or other inspirational literature; choose passages that are encouraging, motivating, comforting. You'll receive a surprising emotional boost from this practice.

8. Before making any major decisions, pray about them, and then listen for God's answer. Read a scriptural passage that might relate to your decision.

Think how this practice has enriched the lives of Steve and Martha Bollinger.

9. Discuss with a beloved and trusted member of the clergy your thoughts about and feelings toward God; many of us have our own unique picture of God that may or may not be emotionally healthy.

I think you'll find that most thoughtful members of the clergy today will emphasize God's infinitely merciful and benevolent nature.

10. Try "stepping-out" in your faith on a regular basis, doing something that in the logical and rational world might seem crazy, but is consistent with your religious principles.

   For example, if you're white, you might want to attend service at an African-American church. If you're Christian, ask a Jewish friend to share Sabbath or a religious holiday meal with your family.

   If you live in the affluent suburbs, attend an inner-city rescue mission and pray with suffering people like Lee Daugherty and Monty Cox.

If You Are Not Religious

1. Keep an open mind to the existence of God and the value of religion or spirituality in your own life and in society. Perhaps discuss God and faith with a religious person whose principles, behavior, and lifestyle you respect and who will accept you without being judgmental.

   It's worth noting that opinion polls show that 96 percent of Americans believe in the existence of God or a higher power.

   As you ponder God's place in the world we can see and touch, bear in mind that cutting-edge scientific disciplines such as molecular biology and astrophysics point increasingly toward order rather than sterile chaos in the universe.

   In June 1998, twenty-seven of the world's leading scientists, including Nobel Prize–winning physicist Charles H. Townes, inventor of the laser, met in Berkeley, California, for a unique seminar, "Science and the Spiritual Quest." Sponsored by the John Templeton Foundation, this first-ever organized effort to reconcile science at the cutting edge with the traditions of monotheistic religion produced a rich interchange of ideas.

   Many of the assembled scientists had never spoken publicly about their faith. But that is changing. Charles Townes told

the group that contemporary scientists are "much more willing
to talk about religion" than they have been in the past.

2. If you've had bad experiences with religion in the past, discuss
them frankly with a religious person you respect. Remember
that religious people have personality problems like everyone
else and often make mistakes or show bad judgment like the
rest of us.

3. Consider attending a church or synagogue as a visitor. Find
one that is "alive" and that actively addresses the needs of the
congregation and today's society. But don't plan only to receive—be ready to give of yourself. Make a sincere effort to get
to know the people in the congregation. Go out to lunch with
them, and take time during the week to call them.

    But it's clear that simply going to church will not make any-
    one religious or spiritual—no more than sitting in your garage
    will turn you into a car.

4. Read the writings of inspired people of deep faith such as C. S.
Lewis; Dr. Albert Schweitzer; Harold Kushner; Martin Luther
King, Jr.; Mother Teresa; and Billy Graham, whose lives exemplify a truly great human spirit worthy of your admiration and
respect.

    Consider reading religious scriptures like the Torah or
    Christian Bible in contemporary versions—for example, *The
    Living Bible* by Tyndale Publishers.

5. Try adapting the suggestions for religious people into your own
situation. From a health perspective, they may work to some
degree for those with few religious or spiritual inclinations.

If You Simply Are Not Yet Ready to Consider Religion

1. Examine the behavior of truly religious/spiritual persons at
your place of work or among your neighbors. Try to emulate
them. Perhaps be generous with your time in helping out and
investing in the lives of others—for example, by defending

and supporting the less fortunate groups in your community.

2. Try nonreligious meditation; this may help you to relax, may convey other health benefits, and may even provide you with religious or spiritual experiences that will increase your interest in finding a place for faith in your life.

3. Honestly reexamine your personal experiences with religion, particularly the negative aspects. Discuss them with a loved and trusted friend who will listen (or, failing that, a professional counselor).

   Many negative religious experiences may stem from an emphasis on such frightening concepts as eternal damnation which see God as judgmental or punishing. Others involve negative interactions with church members or the clergy. Sometimes people have done things they are so ashamed of that they avoid religion because of their guilt. But the spiritually healthy people we've met in this book accentuate the positive, and not the negative. They focus on God's love, kindness, generosity, and forgiveness—seeing all of us as imperfect, and dependent on God's mercy.

Now let's take a look at how these suggestions work in the real world.

The Healing Power of Faith: Jerry Levine, a Living Example

Washington, D.C., real estate attorney Jerry Levine, fifty-three, was raised in a blue-collar, Jewish immigrant home in the old mill town of Meriden, Connecticut. Jerry's grandfather was a tailor, his father a dry cleaner.

"The house was so small," Jerry recalls, "that I slept upstairs with my grandparents."

The Levine women kept a kosher home, and the family observed Sabbath and High Holidays. But for young Jerry, being Jewish in a "one-synagogue town" was more a cultural than a spiritual experience.

For three decades after his bar mitzvah, religion was much less important to him than education and professional achievement.

The first in his family to attend college, Jerry excelled academically,
and did well in law school. He moved to Washington in the 1970s and
began a long apprenticeship learning his complex legal specialty.

Although he wasn't spiritually active, Jerry had never lost the deep
interest in community service that is a hallmark of Judaism. This concern intensified after he married Sarah Pokemaner, a social worker
committed to improving education in crowded District of Columbia
schools. In the mid-1980s, even though he was already overburdened
with a complex and demanding practice, Jerry was drawn toward the
Washington branch of a national volunteer housing rehabilitation
group called Christmas in April. The organization brought churches in
blighted neighborhoods together with volunteers to renovate the
homes of congregation members during a hectic but well-organized
blitz of painting, roofing, carpentry, and plumbing on the last Saturday
of each April.

Jerry led the volunteers from his law firm that first year. They were
assigned a shabby row house on a crack-infested street in northeast
Washington that belonged to a soft-spoken and devout African-American widow. "The Lord will bless you for this," she told Jerry's team as
they struggled with heavy sheets of drywall and scraped paint from the
grimy front porch. Jerry's team worked twelve hours that day, and almost missed the group's celebratory picnic at sunset. But when they left
the home, a collapsed bedroom ceiling and the leaking roof that had
weakened it had been replaced by wallboard and new shingles. The ex-
terior walls had been repainted, and a dangerous, rusty old water heater
replaced by an efficient new gas appliance donated by a local contractor. The team had even cleared the trash from the house's small front
lawn and planted an azalea bush, the optimistic trademark of Christmas in April.

"That experience hooked me," Jerry says. "I realized people coming
together to help on a very basic level could accomplish small miracles."

He immediately volunteered to become a Christmas in April house
captain for the next year. This entailed much more than one day's hard

labor. House captains were responsible to work with volunteer craftsmen to assess the target homes' needs and compile lists of tools and ma-
terials for the specific repairs. Despite this new responsibility, Jerry
became the legal adviser to another community housing group, this one
Jewish.

Yachad ("Unity") combined corporate financial sponsorship with
funding from Washington's large Jewish community to help secure
mortgages for the working poor and other needy families the conventional banking industry usually overlooked.

For the next several years Jerry juggled his legal practice with volunteer work and long hours as a pro bono attorney. In 1991, Yachad sponsored the renovation of a Christmas in April home, donating fifteen
hundred dollars toward supplies.

"Now if we could get some Yachad people to volunteer for work," he
told one of his colleagues.

The man looked slightly embarrassed. "It's on a Saturday, Jerry—
Shabbat," he said.

Jerry was chagrined. In his enthusiasm to ignite the inherent volunteer spirit of the Jewish community, he had forgotten that keeping the
Sabbath was the essence of his religion's spiritual core. Driving into his
office early one morning down Connecticut Avenue, Jerry passed the
large Jewish community center, and the germ of an idea began to form.
There was certainly nothing in the Torah preventing observant Jews
from working on Sundays, the Christian Sabbath. Why couldn't members of synagogues and other Jewish organizations volunteer their time
to renovate homes on the day *after* the Christmas in April teams
worked?

This was the beginning of the organization Sukkoth in April. Jerry and
several friends named their group after the Jewish autumn feast because
it combined the symbolism of harvest shelters with a deeper spiritual significance, the sharing of bounty with the less fortunate. The first year,
1992, Jerry challenged a synagogue to provide both financial sponsorship
and volunteers. Today, sixteen Jewish groups in greater Washington are
working with Sukkoth in April, sharing warehouse space and skilled craft
advice on difficult renovations with the longer-established Christmas in

April. This Jewish volunteer effort is spreading to other cities across the country, thanks in large measure to Jerry Levine's energy and dedication.

During his transformation from a striving young real estate attorney to a middle-age man who now spends fully a third of his year in either pro bono legal or volunteer work, Jerry Levine has also undergone a spiritual metamorphosis.

In 1985, his father, Herman, died, and his and Sarah's oldest daughter, Abigail, was bat mitzvahed. "I think it was more than a midlife crisis," Jerry jokes. "I suddenly felt my own mortality and began asking some big questions: Why was I here? What was the purpose of my life?"

Jerry Levine began attending the large Adas Israel Synagogue, the largest Conservative Jewish congregation in Washington. He started with Sabbath services and slowly expanded his worship practices.

"At first, I just figured this would help me relax," Jerry notes.

Indeed, he found that the tensions of his overcharged week did recede as the rabbi chanted the ancient Hebrew words from the ornate Torah scroll. But soon Jerry found himself seeking a deeper understanding of his faith. He joined religious classes at the synagogue, where he met men his own age who were also embarked on a spiritual quest to explore their religious roots.

Today, Jerry worships at Adas Israel three days a week. He leaves home early each Monday and Thursday morning to join the weekday minyan at the synagogue and spends an hour insulated from the urgency of faxes, E-mail, and legal documents.

"This is *my* time to relax and recharge my soul," Jerry observes. "I may lose an hour's sleep on Monday and Thursday, but I gain a lot more back."

Obviously, Jerry Levine is not alone. The Adas Israel congregation has grown dramatically in recent years. Today there are hundreds of young Jewish families active in the synagogue, many who, like Jerry Levine, felt a hunger that only active faith could satisfy.

I believe that Jerry's use of worship service as a means to "recharge" his spiritual energy goes beyond taking advantage of faith's proven stress-busting attributes. In becoming an active member of the thriving Adas Israel congregation, Jerry Levine has made a connection to an unbroken family and cultural tradition that stretches back, generation by generation, through the millennia to the dawn of recorded history.

When he speaks with pride of young Jewish families working hard to learn the Hebrew of the Torah in order to conduct emotionally powerful services, I believe Jerry is actually describing his own transcendental quest to discover his Jewish roots.

Entering middle age, Jerry is physically healthy and enjoys an abiding sense of inner peace that he probably would have never known had he not cultivated the spiritual side of his nature. Like many fellow Baby Boomers, he has discovered that material success alone and even professional accomplishments linked to volunteer work do not provide the full sense of satisfaction and positive outlook he now enjoys.

"Last Resort" Religion: Shelby's Story, a Life Saved

The painful spiritual journey of one of my patients, a brave woman named Shelby Best, graphically dramatizes that faith can bring healing in even the most seemingly intractable cases of emotional illness.

Shelby, now fifty-six, had suffered from anxiety and depression most of her adult life. She had married young, to an abusive alcoholic who beat her regularly during his binges. In the early 1970s, Shelby, a young woman lacking job skills who had always seen herself as a "fearful person," had been too insecure to leave the relationship. However, her husband left her little choice after she was hospitalized with broken ribs and teeth resulting from his most recent beating.

Back with her parents, Shelby kept her silence as they tried to persuade her to attend church and pray with them, to seek divine help to mend her wounded life. *I won't be a hypocrite*, she thought as her mother brought her a Bible and inspirational books. Although she loved her parents, Shelby had little time for churches. Between binges, her first husband had promised he would turn to religion to help him break the grip of alcohol and adulterous affairs. But he never did. God had not intervened to help then—why would He now?

Shelby was cautiously optimistic when she met Thomas Best, an older, well-spoken ship captain who had been divorced for several years. *Maybe*, she allowed herself to hope, *I might build a life with this good man.*

In fact, Shelby and Thomas were married after a brief courtship and Shelby entered the happiest, most fulfilling years of her life. Thomas was indeed a man worthy of love. Although never truly freed from her chronic anxiety, Shelby did gain enough confidence to look forward to a future with Thomas, a man in whom she was certain she could place her trust. Then one hot July morning in 1985, Shelby Best felt a lump in her right breast and suddenly found herself flung onto the horrifying diagnosis-and-treatment cancer treadmill. As with other forms of modern surgical-medical therapy, the technology had advanced faster than the human dimension of the treatment. Shelby underwent a mastectomy and six months of chemotherapy and received a reconstructive breast implant. The only relief she found for the anxiety that now consumed her was a renewable prescription for a mild tranquilizer.

Convinced that the cancer had spread throughout her body, Shelby sank into depression, with insomnia her worst symptom. Even after her surgeon had assured her he had removed all the cancerous tissue, Shelby found it almost impossible to relax. Five years passed in this fearful state of reprieve until the morning she discovered another lump, this one between the skin of her breast and the implant. Touching the pebble-size bump, she felt a hot flood of terror and bent over, half paralyzed, to vomit. *It's come back to kill me,* she thought, *just like I always knew it would.*

Shelby's second surgery revealed that the cancer had spread to several lymph nodes. She began another regimen of chemotherapy. But even the nausea and weakness associated with the drugs were not as debilitating as her fearful depression. The insomnia returned full force. Her doctors prescribed a stronger tranquilizer, Xanax, which only seemed to worsen her anguish. She then began taking Meprobamate, an even more potent tranquilizer.

On November 6, 1989, two months after her second surgery, Shelby lay tossing on sweaty sheets in her darkened bedroom, battling insomnia for the third night running. Thomas's ship was home in port, but he had gone for a long walk. She suddenly felt a burden of despair simply too heavy to lift. A distant voice seemed to speak inside her mind: *There is only one way the fear will end.*

She turned on the light and groped her way to the dresser, where her medication stood in rows of brown plastic bottles.

"No, no," she mumbled to the disheveled figure in the mirror. "I just can't do this anymore." Then, as she began choking down handfuls of Xanax and Meprobamate caplets, she turned to their dog, Bridgette, sleeping at the foot of the bed and mumbled, "I'm *so* sorry."

When Thomas returned an hour later, he found Shelby lying on the floor, near death, surrounded by empty prescription bottles.

Shelby regained consciousness strapped to a bed in a psychiatric hospital, the room lit around the clock as the staff kept her under suicide watch. She chewed her food and took her medications, trying to build the plausible facade of a compliant patient. But inside the chill voice still spoke, reminding her there was only *one* way to leave her pain behind.

Her first chance came after a few days when she discovered that a patient had left a pair of panty hose to dry in the shower stall.

Shelby twisted the stretchy fabric into a clumsy noose and had already blacked out before the orderlies cut her down and removed the hose from her bleeding neck. Another day, she staggered groggily from her bed and thrust her face deep into the toilet bowl, choking on the water as she tried unsuccessfully to drown herself. Then she found a sliver of glass in a flower bed and used it to slit her wrists.

The doctors and orderlies finally lost patience. Shelby spent thirty-eight days in the acute psychiatric ward, many of them strapped in a straitjacket inside a dim, padded cell, the panic building to intolerable levels.

Finally, a physician who was a family friend with deep religious conviction and Shelby's attorney intervened to have her transferred to the 3 East psychiatric unit at Duke University Medical Center. My colleague, psychiatrist Dr. Andrea Allen, took over Shelby's care. After several weeks of detoxification from the heavy doses of tranquilizers and antidepressants she'd been on, Shelby began electroconvulsive therapy.

She was released home in 1990. But few of the doctors who had treated her were optimistic about her prognosis.

Then, almost on an impulse, Shelby agreed to join friends one Sunday morning at church. It would be nice and very convenient to report a sudden and dramatic conversion-healing experience, but the reality of Shelby's case is almost as compelling. After a few Sundays, she found herself looking forward to attending service, as much to hear the comforting old hymns of her childhood as to receive any message of redemption. But, several months after her release from the hospital, Shelby had also begun to pray, tentatively at first, then fervently, both at church and alone at home.

One morning when Thomas was gone and she was busy in the kitchen, she looked up from the sink, seized by a revelation more powerful than any of her paralytic fears had ever been.

"*I* was the one who left God," she whispered. "He never left me. Praise the Lord. Thank you, Jesus."

From that morning on, Shelby made a conscious effort to increase the role of faith in her life. She became more active in her church and studied scripture privately.

A steady improvement occurred in her mood and thinking. This was surprising, given her previous condition and the fact that she was off all medication except for a relatively minor antidepressant.

"What did you *do* that helped so much?" I later asked.

"I tried to focus more on God than on myself," Shelby answered.

There was certainly very little in the psychiatric therapy texts I'd studied to help me evaluate the efficacy of such spiritual healing. But I continued to see steady progress in Shelby.

Her new stability was soon put to a severe test. Thomas's son from his first marriage, Leonard, returned home from New York, where he had followed his father's seagoing tradition and taken work as a tugboat captain. But Leonard was also from a generation that took more risks: He had become infected with HIV through injecting drugs. He now had AIDS.

Thomas never stopped loving his son, but could not bear the strain of watching the once-handsome and muscular young man wither away. The burden of Leonard's care fell on Shelby.

These two wounded people bonded closely and helped each other heal emotionally. I don't mean that Leonard was miraculously cured of AIDS; in fact he died, his body scourged by the disease, in September 1994. But he achieved an inner peace before his death. And, as Shelby helped him, she gained some of his courage, which gave her confidence to face the rest of her life.

In nursing the young man through the pain and disfigurement of the terrible opportunistic infections that follow AIDS, Shelby was able to put her own humanity and mortality into perspective. Watching Leonard accept the inevitable approach of his death with grace and even humor, Shelby was finally freed of the death anxiety that had stalked her for years.

"Shelby," Leonard weakly told her one grim night after almost slipping away to toxoplasmosis, "don't worry about me. I'm going to be all right."

She realized that Leonard's body was dying, practically before her eyes, but also that he had come to recognize that the disease could not touch his soul.

On good days, Shelby took Leonard on outings down to the ocean, where she could push his wheelchair along the boardwalk between the dunes, he could wade in the surf, and they could watch the seagulls and fishing boats.

"God sure has created a beautiful world," Leonard told her.

For the first time in years, Shelby was able to see that beauty.

When death finally freed Leonard from his pain, Shelby was surprised to sense a solid core of optimism under her grief. She was absolutely certain that the young man now resided in a better place beyond the grave.

Her stability was tested once more fourteen months later when Thomas died of cancer only seven months after being diagnosed with terminal illness. Again, Shelby was assaulted by the essence of her worst nightmares—relentless, stalking death. I have no doubt that this trauma once would have driven her back into suicidal depression. But her newfound religious faith shielded her, allowing Shelby to cope.

Although she had returned to religion as an adult fighting a desperate and seemingly hopeless struggle against mental illness, Shelby now embraced her faith with a calm maturity. Again, she realized that God had always been in her life, even though she had not been able to see His presence.

"God directed me to the right doctors," she told me. "He has allowed me to finally see that I am a very strong person. Whatever happens to my body, I know I have Jesus, and that He's never going to leave me. I have felt the touch of the Master's hand."

Today, Shelby Best works as a volunteer with HOPE, a support group for people who have encountered devastating illness, either their own or in loved ones. She is able to recognize and soothe the sense of anguished hopelessness that so often blights the lives of people confronting serious disease.

"You are not alone in this struggle," she tells them. "For years I thought I was alone, but I was wrong. God was watching. I tried to take my life many times, but He wouldn't let me. He always gave me another chance. Now He has given me wisdom and insight that I never thought possible. He can do the same for you."

Although Shelby Best turned to religion almost by accident and as a last resort, it is clear to me that she has benefited from the healing power of faith to a degree and in a manner that medical science would once not have found credible. We can all learn from Shelby Best's spiritual journey.

Harnessing the Power of Faith for Loved Ones' Health

As I noted earlier, there are people who lack religious faith but are willing to expand their spiritual lives, and there are others who sincerely feel they are not yet ready to consider religion. You may find yourself in either of these categories, but with a loved one who *is* religious and whose emotional or physical health could benefit from the healing power of faith, as we've discussed that process in this book. Is there any practical way that you, a nonbeliever, can form a spiritual connection with a religious loved one? I am confident that there is.

Sandra's Story

Consider the touching story of Sandra, an intelligent, well-educated, and successful New York publishing executive who never nurtured the spiritual roots of her Judaism. A morally upright and conscientious person with a strong sense of social justice, Sandra was born into an assimilated intellectual family in which girls were not encouraged to take an interest in faith, beyond the minimum cultural conventions of observing High Holidays. She went through college and entered professional life involved in the civil rights movement, but without much curiosity about transcendental matters.

Then one afternoon a few years ago, she received a frantic phone call at her office. Her father had suffered a serious heart attack and had been rushed to the intensive care unit of a suburban hospital. Almost numb with anguish, she grabbed her purse and turned toward the office door, debating whether a taxi or the subway would be her fastest route through the rush-hour traffic to the hospital.

Her phone rang, and Sandra considered not answering, but finally snatched up the receiver impatiently. "Did you hear the terrible news?" It was her uncle Aaron, her father's older brother, a kindly man who had become increasingly religious as he matured.

"I'm on my way to the hospital now," Sandra said, suppressing any hint of impatience.

But Aaron insisted on talking. "I contacted Jonathan in Israel," he said, referring to his son, who lived near Jerusalem. "He's on his way to the Western Wall to pray for your father."

As was her habit, Sandra scrawled a note on the yellow pad and tore off the page. "Thanks . . . that's very kind." She jammed the page into her purse. "Uncle Aaron, I've got to go."

At the hospital, Sandra, normally a thorough and decisive person, felt helpless as the doctors and nurses worked on her father, who lay, his naked chest plastered with sensor pads, amid a web of tubes and wires strung between gleaming equipment.

Sandra alternated between abject depression that her father was slipping inexorably away and groundless optimism that *somehow* all this medical high technology would save him.

She forgot about the scrawled note in her purse. And she did not request a visit from the rabbinical chaplain. Later that long night, when a nurse suggested it might be time for the rabbi to come and pray, Sandra rejected the idea because such a deathbed vigil would have dashed the last of her remaining optimism.

Sandra's father died less than a day after being admitted. He never had the comfort of knowing that his nephew Jonathan was praying for his salvation with other devout men at the ancient wall in Jerusalem that is Judaism's holiest site. Nor did he experience the spiritual warmth of prayer in his final hours.

Looking back at this experience, Sandra feels a sense of regret, but sees that we can all learn a lesson from her father's death. "Even though I am not religious myself," she says, "I definitely should have mentioned that Jonathan was praying for him. That would have brought Dad comfort."

She adds that prayer from a rabbinical chaplain might have depressed her, but that the prayers would have bolstered her father's spirits. Now, Sandra suggests to Jewish friends her age that, even if they personally lack faith, they can take active steps to avoid the mistakes she made. In the event of a loved one's hospitalization, she advises, they can:

- Contact the person's congregation and ask the rabbi to pray for recovery. And—most important—they can inform the person these prayers are being said.
- Request, if the family has religious relatives in Israel, that they pray for the patient at the Wall, and inform the patient of these prayers.
- Arrange for regular rabbinical chaplain visits to the hospitalized patient.

• Encourage religious friends and relatives to visit the hospital, bringing messages of faith.

Sandra emphasizes that none of these activities are incompatible with anyone's system of belief, be it faith or skepticism. But, again, the spiritual and emotional bolstering the hospitalized patient receives can only be beneficial.

Further Steps for the Nonbeliever to Help a Religious Loved One Who Is Ill

Sandra's concrete suggestions on "focusing" spirituality during a health crisis certainly apply to all monotheistic religions. With this in mind, you may want to consider the following steps in a similar situation.

1. Contact your loved one's clergy and ask them to say special prayers or perform a religious ritual for the ill person. For Roman Catholics, you may wish to dedicate a mass. For Protestants, request special congregational prayers to be said during service. Many Jewish congregations will also say special prayers for the recovery of the ill. Jewish healing centers will send spiritual counselors to visit your ill loved one. Be sure to tell the patient what you have done, not to claim credit, but to extend emotional solidarity.

2. If the ill person has faith in religious shrines or sites (Lourdes, the Western Wall, etc.), request that prayers for their recovery be said there.

3. Give the person an inspirational book, audio book, or CD with religious music. This might provide comfort during periods of lonely anguish.

4. Take an active role in assuring that a chaplain or member of the clergy regularly visits and prays with your loved one, whether the patient is hospitalized or being treated at home. Ask the clergy member to inform your loved one of your interest in this

matter. This will also demonstrate spiritual solidarity.

5. Help collect and deliver to the hospital messages of faith from members of your loved one's religious community and from religious friends and relatives.

6. If your loved one is convalescing, offer transportation to attend religious services. If the patient has hearing or visual impairment, you can arrange for adaptive devices: scripture or other inspirational literature in large-print editions (*Guidepost* for the Christian) or audio book versions of the Bible, with a tape cassette player. You might consider arranging for cable TV at the hospital so your loved one can watch the Inspirational Channel while recuperating.

7. If your loved one's health is stable and you simply want to provide the healing benefits of faith, consider offering tickets to a religious play, concert of sacred music, or religious lecture or seminar, or even underwriting a religious pilgrimage.

8. Consider attending religious services *with* your loved one. Remember, nonbelievers attend weddings and funerals, so your participating in religious services with loved ones is more about *their* faith and *your* love than about your actual conversion.

9. Offer a financial donation to your loved ones' church or synagogue as a symbol of your respect for their faith.

10. If your loved one has a religious younger relative, you might offer to pay for the child's attendance at a religious school, summer camp, or retreat. Again, this will demonstrate your respect for the role of religion in your loved one's life.

11. Unless you are an inflexible atheist, you might consider telling your loved one, "*If* there is a God, then I pray to that God for your health and well-being." This shows your loved one that you are keeping an open mind, which can be seen as an important act of compassion by the religious person.

Final Thoughts

Looking back fifteen years, I vividly recall my morning ward rounds, when I first noticed that several patients were praying or reading scripture. That was when I began to wonder what influence faith might have on their ability to cope with health problems. Now I am amazed at what science has discovered about the wide-ranging effects that devout religious faith and practice may have on mental and physical health and on quality of life for individuals, families, and communities. Almost every area of life and health appears to be affected by deep religious faith that is lived within in a community of believers. In summing up this book, I would like to emphasize several important points.

- First, I believe that it takes both a deep personal faith in God and active involvement in a faith community for people to obtain maximum health benefits. Neither a strong personal faith practiced in isolation (private meditation, study, or devotion without connection or service to others) or active church or synagogue attendance without a deep personal faith (service to others in the absence of belief) will achieve the benefits that combining faith and religious involvement will.

  Helen Koebert and her sisters in Milwaukee exemplify the blending of a deep personal commitment with a living testament of that commitment through service to their church and community.
- Second, if the sole intention of belief or worship service is to obtain health benefits, it is likely that better health will not result. For that would be an "extrinsic" use of religion—religion as a means to another end, rather than as an end in itself. Such a manipulation of faith has actually been correlated with worse health and greater unhappiness. If you include religion in your life from a sincere sense of faith, better mental and physical health may naturally follow. This has clearly been the experience of Walter and Marguerite Grounds, whose whole lives have always been centered on their faith.

• Third, sickness, poor health, and even emotional illness do not necessarily mean a weak faith. I have known many people with very serious medical or psychiatric illnesses whose faith and spiritual endurance I have greatly admired. Certainly Khalita Jones is gravely ill, but spiritually healthy. And disease has ravaged Genie Lewis's body, but her spirit is robust. It is their faith and trust in God that has literally kept them alive. Telling people who are already carrying such heavy burdens that their illness stems from weak faith can be very damaging, bringing them doubt and undercutting their ability to use their faith as a resource. Encouragement and support is what such persons need, not criticism or a sanctimonious attitude.

• Fourth, many of the research studies reviewed and personal stories told in this book have involved older people. Some of you may wonder what relevance all of this has for younger persons. But for younger people like Chris Benfield, Khalita Jones, and Dan and Marcia, it is clear that faith played an instrumental role in shaping their lives. Further, our Duke research and that of others, such as the landmark studies led by Strawbridge and Kark, suggest that the health benefits of faith and religious involvement are not only experienced by the elderly, but by younger people as well. In fact, given that younger people have so much more of their lives to live, it is likely that the health benefits of a strong faith accumulate over the years and thus may have even greater consequences for them. This is particularly true for adolescents, when delinquency, suicide, drugs, and dangerous sexual practices threaten to destroy lives that are just beginning.

• Fifth, let's review what I mean when I speak of religion and faith. What religion? Faith in what? There is now scientific evidence suggesting that the "content" of faith can make a difference in its healing consequences.[1] On the one hand, a belief system will probably have positive health effects if it presents God as all-powerful, personal, responsive, loving, just, forgiving, immensely merciful, and understanding. This kind of God encourages love and service and is rooted in an established religious tradition whose leaders are held accountable to others. On the other hand, health benefits are ultimately less likely to come from a belief system that sees God as punishing, angry, vengeful, and distant; that encourages unthinking, unquestioning devotion and obedience to a single leader who has absolute power and lacks accountability; and that isolates members from their families and larger community.

Patient-Centered Prayer

What are the implications of the exciting new research findings we've presented in this book for the practice of medicine? Should doctors actually *prescribe* belief in God, regular churchgoing, prayer, and daily reading of the scriptures? Should doctors pray with every patient?

I would not suggest any of these things. What I am suggesting is a more sensitive, patient-centered approach. First, all physicians and health professionals should take a religious history from their patients. If the health professional feels comfortable addressing religious or spiritual questions, then I think it's proper to let the patient know it is permissible to discuss them.

In certain circumstances where religion might be of particular comfort to a believing patient, as in situations of severe pain, great suffering, terminal illness, poor prognosis, loss of a loved one, presurgery, or severe chronic stress, the health professional might ask the patient if prayer would be helpful. In such a situation I suggest that the patient do the praying and the health professional participate by saying "Amen." If the patient wishes, the health professional may lead a short prayer.

Patients should feel free to bring up spiritual or religious issues with their doctors, particularly if they feel uncomfortable discussing such issues with their minister or chaplain. Talking about religious and spiritual matters is almost always most comfortable if patient and physician have a similar religious background.

Another way to integrate the healing power of faith into health care is by including a chaplain on the hospitalized patient's care team, who can join the physicians and nurses every morning on rounds. This is now being done at major hospitals in the Midwest, and, as Rev. Brenda Peterson's story has shown, in California. Further, the parish nurse program is an excellent way of providing congregations with health professionals who are members of the faith community and who can screen for medical problems such as high blood pressure or diabetes, diagnose illness and refer congregants to specialists in a timely manner, provide health education, and monitor patients for compliance with treatment.

Finally, I would like to emphasize once again what I mean by "healing." Healing can include dramatic, sudden physical cures, but is not confined to the "miraculous" or the spectacular. Perhaps for most people, the healing power of faith involves a healing of the mind and emotions, of the intangible spirit, and of relationships with others. In the end, achieving this type of inner peace may or may not result in physical healing; but even if the physical is not healed, it is very likely the burden of illness will be lighter. Such healings may be sudden, or they can take time—often months, sometimes years. Faith often involves persistence and patience. Faith is confidence that you will receive what you desire before you actually have it. Faith involves a kind of positive thinking that by itself heals and prepares the body for healing. Most of the true angst and suffering that people experience is not a result of physical pain, but of outlook, emotions, and relationships with others. Healing in these areas can put physical health problems in true perspective, prevent them from dominating our lives, liberate us from stress and depression, and free the body to heal itself.

This has clearly been the experience of Khalita Jones, who has decided to focus her attention on God and spiritual matters, allowing her physical healing to take a lower priority than her relationship with God. For the chronically ill, the search for physical healing can often become an unobtainable idol in their lives. Faith can put that physical illness beneath us, where it belongs, return dominion to us, and give us power to live victorious and fulfilled lives.

Faith on Medicine's Frontier

I firmly believe that we are on the brink of a great new era in medicine: a time when health professionals will begin to help people regain control over their lives by providing them with the spiritual tools to maintain health and wellness, and thus enable them to take maximum advantage of the healing power that faith can give us all.

Notes

Chapter One: Science, Religion, and Health

1. Nila Kirkpatrick Covalt, M.D. "The Meaning of Religion to Older People," *Geriatrics* (September 1960): 659.
2. Harold G. Koenig, "Religious Behaviors and Death Anxiety in Later Life," *The Hospice Journal* 4, no. 1 (1988): 3.
3. George H. Gallup, Jr., *Religion in America 1996* (Princeton, NJ: The Princeton Religion Research Center, 1996), 4, 12, 19.

Chapter Two: Faith and Life Satisfaction

1. Harold G. Koenig, James N. Kvale, and Carolyn Ferrel. "Religion and Well-Being in Later Life," *The Gerontologist* 28 (1988): 18–28.
2. For more information on this medical school curriculum grant program, contact John Templeton Foundation, P.O. Box 8322, Radnor, PA 19087-8322.
3. H. G. Koenig, L. K. George, and B. L. Peterson. "Religiosity and Remission from Depression in Medically Ill Older Patients," *American Journal of Psychiatry* 155 (1998): 536–42.
4. The following sources provide a representative sample of Benson's work on this fascinating subject. Herbert Benson, M.D., *Timeless Healing, The Power of Biology and Belief* (New York: Simon & Schuster, 1997), 115–20, 243–44; Herbert Benson, M.D., "The Relaxation Response: Its Subjective and Objective Historical Precedents and Physiology," *TINS*

6 (1983): 281–84; Herbert Benson, M.D., S. Alexander, and C. L. Feldman, "Decreased Premature Ventricular Contractions Through Use of Relaxation Response in Patients with Stable Ischemic Heart Disease," *The Lancet* 2 (1975): 380–82.

5. Gordon W. Allport, *The Individual and His Religion: A Psychological Interpretation* (New York: Macmillan, 1950); Gordon W. Allport and J. M. Ross. "Personal Religious Orientation and Prejudice," *Journal of Personality and Social Psychology* 5 (1967): 432–43.

6. Koenig et al. "Religion and Well-Being in Later Life," 22–26. The Duke University Center for the Study of Religion/Spirituality and Health currently uses the following statements to determine a person's degree of intrinsic religiosity: "In my life, I experience the presence of the Divine (i.e., God)"; "My religious beliefs are what really lie behind my whole approach to life"; "I try hard to carry my religion over into all other dealings in life." Research subjects can answer on the following scale: "Definitely true of me"; "Tends to be true"; "Unsure"; "Tends *not* to be true"; "Definitely *not* true." For more information see: H. G. Koenig, K. G. Meador, and G. Parkerson. "Religion Index for Psychiatric Research," *American Journal of Psychiatry* 154 (1997): 885–86.

7. H. G. Koenig, D. O. Moberg, and J. N. Kvale. "Religious Activities and Attitudes of Older Adults in a Geriatric Assessment Clinic," *Journal of the American Geriatric Society* 36 (1988): 362–74.

8. U.S. Department of Health and Human Services, *Physical Activity and Health, A Report of the Surgeon General* (U.S. Department of Health and Human Services, Centers for Disease Control and Prevention, National Center for Chronic Disease Prevention and Health Promotion, 1996), 81–172.

9. Christopher G. Ellison. "Religious Involvement and Subjective Well-Being," *Journal of Health and Social Behavior* 32 (March 1991): 90.

10. Ibid., 89.

11. Jeffrey S. Levin, Linda M. Chatters, and Robert Joseph Taylor. "Religious Effects on Health Status and Life Satisfaction Among Black Americans," *Journal of Gerontology: Social Sciences* 50B, no. 3 (1995): 158–61.

12. J. S. Levin, K. S. Markides, and L. A. Ray. "Religious Attendance and

Psychological Well-Being in Mexican Americans: A Panel Analysis of Three Generations' Data," *The Gerontologist* 36 (1996): 454–63. See also: J. S. Levin and K. S. Markides. "Religious Attendance and Psychological Well-Being in Middle-Aged and Older Mexican Americans," *Sociological Analysis* 49 (1988): 66–72.

13. P. J. Handal, W. Black-Lopez, S. Moergen. "Preliminary Investigation of the Relationship Between Religion and Psychological Distress in Black Women," *Psychological Reports* 65 (1989): 971–75.

Chapter Three: Religious People Have Stronger Marriages and Families

1. National Center for Health Statistics, *Monthly Vital Statistics Report* 45, no. 12 (July 17, 1997); see also vol. 46, no. 6 (January 28, 1998).

2. National Center for Health Statistics, *Monthly Vital Statistics Report* 43, no. 9(S) (March 22, 1995).

3. Nicholas Zill and Charlotte A. Schoenborn. "Developmental, Learning, and Emotional Problems: Health of Our Nation's Children, United States, 1988," *Advance Data*, National Center for Health Statistics, no. 190 (November 16, 1990): 1–18.

4. Ibid, p. 8.

5. Nicholas Zill, D. R. Morrison, and M. J. Coiro. "Long-Term Effects of Parental Divorce on Parent-Child Relationships, Adjustment, and Achievement in Young Adulthood," *Journal of Family Psychology* 7, no. 1 (1993): 96.

6. W. Shrum. "Religion and Marital Instability: Change in the 1970s," *Review of Religious Research* 212 (1980): 135–47.

7. Kenneth I. Pargament, *The Psychology of Religion and Coping* (New York: The Guildford Press, 1997), 179. See also: M. R. Wilson and E. E. Filsinger. "Religiosity and Marital Adjustment: Multidimensional Interrelationships," *Journal of Marriage and the Family* 48 (February 1986): 147–51.

8. L. C. Robinson. "Religious Orientation in Enduring Marriage: An

Exploratory Study," *Review of Religious Research* 35, no. 3 (March 1994): 207–9.

9. Every established religious organization in the United States and Canada now provides some form of organized marital counseling, generally available through local churches and synagogues. One of the most thorough and successful is the Retrouvaille ("Rediscovery") program of the Roman Catholic Church. From my experience, marital counseling that draws on a couple's religious faith works from a firmer foundation than purely secular counseling. This is because, ultimately, the couple share some degree of spiritual certainty, while they often disagree on other major life values.

10. Philip R. Kunz and Stan L. Albrecht. "Religion, Marital Happiness, and Divorce," *International Journal of Sociology of the Family* 7 (1977): 230.

11. W. R. Schumm, S. R. Bollman, and A. P. Jurich. "The 'Marital Conventionalization' Argument: Implications for the Study of Religiosity and Marital Satisfaction," *Journal of Psychology and Theology* 10, no. 3 (1982): 236–41.

12. Jeremy D. Kark, Galia Shemi, Yechiel Friedlander, Oz Martin, Orly Manor, and S. H. Blondheim. "Does Religious Observance Promote Health? Mortality in Secular vs. Religious Kibbutzim in Israel," *American Journal of Public Health* 86, no. 3 (March 1996): 345–46.

13. Margaret R. Wilson and Erik E. Filsinger. "Religiosity and Marital Adjustment: Multidimensional Inter-relationships," *Journal of Marriage and the Family* 48 (February 1986): 150.

14. C. L. Shehan, E. W. Bock, and G. R. Lee. "Religious Heterogamy, Religiosity, and Marital Happiness: The Case of Catholics," *Journal of Marriage and the Family* 52 (1990): 77.

15. M. G. Dudley and F. A. Kosinski. "Religiosity and Marital Satisfaction: A Research Note," *Review of Religious Research* 32, no. 1 (1990): 78–86.

16. Howard Weinberg. "Marital Reconciliation in the United States: Which Couples Are Successful?" *Journal of Marriage and the Family* (February 1994): 86.

17. L. C. Robinson. "Religious Orientation in Enduring Marriage: An Exploratory Study," *Review of Religious Research* 35 (1994): 211.

18. "Covenant Marriage Act: Contracting a Covenant Marriage," pam-

phlet provided by the State of Louisiana, Department of Justice, P.O. Box 94095, Baton Rouge, LA 70804, referring to the Covenant Marriage Act, LSA-R.S. 9:272, et seq.

Chapter Four: Religious People Have Healthy Lifestyles

1. Researchers unfamiliar with contemporary and scripturally based Islamic health concepts will find information in this book: Abdulfattah O. A. Olayiwola, *Health Science in Islam* (Lagos, Nigeria, Al-Tawheed Publishers, 1991).

2. P. H. Hardestym and K. M. Kirby. "Relation Between Family Religiousness and Drug Use Within Adolescent Peer Groups," *Journal of Social Behavior and Personality* 10, no. 1 (1995): 421–30.

3. M. J. Donahue and P. L. Benson. "Religion and the Well-Being of Adolescents," *Journal of Social Issues* 51, no. 2 (1995): 153.

4. F. Alexander and R. W. Duff. "Influence of Religiosity and Alcohol Use on Personal Well-being," *Journal of Religious Gerontology* 8, no. 2 (1991): 11–21.

5. H. G. Koenig, D. O. Moberg, and J. N. Kvale. "Religious Activities and Attitudes of Older Adults in a Geriatric Assessment Clinic," *Journal of the American Geriatric Society* 36 (1988): 366.

6. D. P. Desmond and J. F. Maddux. "Religious Programs and Careers of Chronic Heroin Users," *American Journal of Drug and Alcohol Abuse* 8, no. 1 (1981): 71–83.

7. D. P. Desmond and J. F. Maddux, "Religious Programs and Careers of Chronic Heroin Users."

8. For a summary of this study, see: Dale A. Matthews, David B. Larson, Constance P. Barry, *The Faith Factor: An Annotated Bibliography of Clinical Research on Spiritual Subjects*, vol. 1 (Rockville, MD, National Institute for Healthcare Research, 1993), 72–3.

9. D. Hasin, J. Endicott, and C. Lewis. "Alcohol and Drug Use in Patients with Affective Syndromes." *Comprehensive Psychiatry* 26, no. 3 (1985): 283–95.

10. George E. Valliant, M.D., *The Natural History of Alcoholism: Causes, Patterns, and Paths to Recovery* (Cambridge, MA: Harvard University Press, 1983).

11. George E. Valliant, M.D., *The Natural History of Alcoholism*.

12. For an insightful discussion of the power of religious faith to break addiction, see: Pargament, *The Psychology of Religion and Coping*, 147–49; 393–97.

13. H. G. Koenig, L. K. George, K. G. Meador, D. G. Blazer, and S. M. Ford. "Religious practices and Alcoholism in a Southern Adult Population," *Hospital & Community Psychiatry* 45 (1994): 225–31.

14. Ibid., 230–31.

15. M. Galanter. "Religious Conversions: An Experimental Model for Affecting Alcoholic Denial," *Currents in Alcoholism* 6 (1979): 69–78, 1979.

16. Ruth's story is told in a brief unpublished memoir, *A Spiritual Awakening*, graciously provided by Maxine Uttal, director, Jewish Alcoholics, Chemically Dependent Persons and Significant Others (JACS). Persons wishing more information on this innovative program should write to JACS, 426 W. 58th St., New York, NY 10011; telephone: 212-397-4197; fax: 212-489-6229; E-mail: jacs@jacsweb.org.

17. I. Waldron. "The Contribution of Smoking to Sex Differences in Mortality," *Public Health Report* 101 (1986): 163–73.

18. H. G. Koenig, L. K. George, H. J. Cohen, J. C. Hays, D. B. Larson, and D. G. Blazer. "The Relationship Between Religious Activities and Cigarette Smoking in Older Adults," *Journal of Gerontology* (medical sciences) 53A (1998): M426–M434.

19. S. R. Burkett. "Religion, Parental Influence, and Adolescent Alcohol and Marijuana Use," *Journal of Drug Issues* 7, no. 3 (1977): 263–73.

20. A. V. Amoateng, and S. J. Bahr. "Religion, Family and Adolescent Drug Use," *Sociological Perspectives* 29, no. 1 (1986): 53–76. E. M. Adlaf and R. G. Smart. "Drug Use and Religious Affiliation: Feelings and Behavior," *British Journal of Addiction* 80 (1985): 163–71.

21. K. S. Kendler, C. O. Gardner, and C. A. Prescott. "Religion, Psychopathology, and Substance Use and Abuse: A Multimeasure, Genetic-Epidemiologic Study," *American Journal of Psychiatry* 154 (March

3, 1997): 322–27. Also see: S. R. Burkett. "Perceived Parents' Religiosity, Friends' Drinking, and Hellfire: A Panel Study of Alcoholic Drinking," *Review of Religious Research* 35 (1993): 134–53.

22. Centers for Disease Control and Prevention et al., *Physical Activity and Health, A Report of the Surgeon General* (Washington, D.C., U.S. Department of Health and Human Services, 1997), 133.

23. L. F. Berkman and S. L. Syme. "Social Networks, Host Resistance, and Mortality: A Nine-Year Follow-up Study of Alameda County Residents," *American Journal of Epidemiology* 109 (1979): 186–204.

24. Carole Lewis, with W. Terry Whalin, *First Place: The Original Spiritually Based Weight Loss Plan for Whole Person Fitness* (Nashville: Broadman & Holdman Publishers, 1998).

25. Dana Hull. "Dieters Putting Their Faith in Sustenance of the Spirit," *Washington Post*, May 17, 1997, C6. Linus Mundy, *The Complete Guide to Prayer Walking: A Simple Path to Body-&-Soul Fitness* (St. Meinrad, IN: Abbey Press, 1997).

26. People seeking more information on this program should write to: The International Parish Nurse Resource Center, 205 W. Touhy Avenue, Suite 104, Park Ridge, IL 60068-1174.

27. Pargament, *The Psychology of Religion and Coping*, 323–29.

28. C. Spence, T. S. Danielson, and W. M. Kaunitz. "The Faith Assembly: A Study of Perinatal and Maternal Mortality," *Indiana Medicine* (March 1984): 180–83. And: C. Spence and T. S. Danielson. "The Faith Assembly: A Follow-Up Study of Faith Healing and Mortality," *Indiana Medicine* (March 1987): 238–40.

29. M. A. E. Conyn-van Spaendonck, P. M. Oostvogel, A. M. van Loon, et al. "Circulation of Poliovirus During the Poliomyelitis Outbreak in the Netherlands, in 1992–1993," *American Journal of Epidemiology* 143 (1996): 929–35.

30. S. M. Asser and R. Swan. "Child Fatalities From Religion-Motivated Medical Neglect," *Pediatrics* 101, no. 4 (April 1998): 625–29.

31. *60 Minutes*, February 1, 1998; transcript copyright 1998, Dow Jones & Company, Inc.

Chapter Five: Religious People Cope Well with Stress

1. R. Blum. "Contemporary Threats to Adolescent Health in the United States," *Journal of the American Medical Association* 257, no. 24 (June 26, 1987): 3390–95.

2. Peter Davies, Ph.D. "Confronting Alzheimer's: New Gains on an Elusive Enemy," *1989 Medical and Health Annual* (Chicago: Encyclopaedia Britanic, 1990), 186, 201.

3. S. Wright, C. Pratt, and V. Schmall. "Spiritual Support for Caregivers of Dementia Patients," *Journal of Religion and Health* 24, no. 1 (1985): 31–8.

4. K. I. Mation. "The Stress-Buffering Role of Spiritual Support: Cross-Sectional and Prospective Investigation," *Journal for the Scientific Study of Religion* 28, no. 3 (1989): 310–23.

5. Ibid., p. 320.

6. H. G. Koenig, L. K. George, and I. C. Siegler. "The Use of Religion and Other Emotion-Regulating Coping Strategies Among Older Adults," *Gerontologist* 28, no. 3 (1988): 303–10.

7. Nila K. Covalt. "The Meaning of Religion to Older People," 659.

8. H. G. Koenig, H. J. Cohen, D. G. Blazer, C. Pieper, K. G. Meador, et al. "Religious Coping and Depression in Elderly Hospitalized Medically Ill Men," *American Journal of Psychiatry* 149 (1992): 1693–1700.

9. H. G. Koenig. "Religious Attitudes and Practices of Hospitalized Medically Ill Older Adults," *International Journal of Geriatric Psychiatry* 13 (1998): 213–24.

10. Koenig et al. "Religious Coping and Depression in Elderly Hospitalized Medically Ill Men," *American Journal of Psychiatry* 149 (1992): 1693–1700.

11. H. G. Koenig, et al. "Use of Religion by Patients with Severe Medical Illness," *Mind/Body Medicine* 2, no. 1 (1997): 31–6.

12. Kenneth I. Pargament, *The Psychology of Religion and Coping* (New York: The Guildford Press, 1997). Chapter Seven, "The Many Faces of Religion in Coping," pp. 163–97, is especially illuminating.

13. K. I. Pargament, Davis S. Ensing, Kathryn Falgout, Hannah Olsen, Barbara Reilly, Kimberly Van Haitsma, and Richard Warren. "God Help

Me (I): Religious Coping Efforts as Predictors of the Outcomes to Significant Negative Life Events," *American Journal of Community Psychology* 18, no. 6 (1990): 793–824.

14. Ibid., 14.

15. Neal Krause and Thanh Van Tran. "Stress and Religious Involvement Among Older Blacks," *Journal of Gerontology, Social Sciences* 44, no. 1 (1989): S4–13.

16. National Center for Health Statistics, *Monthly Vital Statistics Report* 45, no. 11 (5)2, June 12, 1997; Table 7, 24.

17. R. Blum, "Contemporary Threats to Adolescent Health in the United States," *Journal of the American Medical Association* 257, no. 24 (June 26, 1987): 3390–95.

18. Martin E. P. Seligman. "Optimism, Hope, and Ending the Epidemic of Depression," Symposium, the John Templeton Foundation, February 10, 1998. Also: Martin E. P. Seligman, *The Optimistic Child* (Boston: Houghton Mifflin Co., 1995).

19. M. J. Donahue and P. L. Benson. "Religion and the Well-Being of Adolescents," *Journal of Social Issues* 51, no. 2 (1995): 145–60.

20. Ibid., 149.

21. Ibid., 157.

Chapter Six: Religion Offers Protection from Depression and Helps Those Afflicted to Recover Quickly

1. H. A. Pincus, et al. "Prescribing Trends in Psychotropic Medications, Primary Care, Psychiatry, and Other Medical Specialties," *Journal of the American Medical Association* 279, no. 7 (February 18, 1998): 530.

2. "Antidepressant Prescriptions Soar as Tranquilizers Fall," *Washington Post*, February 19, 1998, A8.

3. National Institute of Mental Health, "Facts About Depression," Internet information: WWW.NIMH.NIH.GOV, April 4, 1998.

4. H. G. Koenig, K. G. Meador, H. J. Cohen, and D. G. Blazer. "Depression in Elderly Patients Hospitalized with Medical Illness," *Archives of Internal Medicine* 148, 1929–36.

5. Paul Cowan, *An Orphan in History* (Garden City, New York: Doubleday, 1982).

6. Hirshel Jaffe, James Rudin, and Marcia Rudin, *Why Me? Why Anyone?* (New York: St. Martin's Press, 1986).

7. S. J. M. Fernando. "A Cross-Cultural Study of Some Familial and Social Factors in Depressive Illness," *British Journal of Psychiatry* 127 (1975): p. 51. Also: S. J. M. Fernando. "Aspects of Depression in a Jewish Minority Group," *Psychiatria Clinica* 11 (1978): 23–33.

8. J. A. Cook and D. W. Wimberley. "If I Should Die Before I Wake: Religious Commitment and Adjustment to the Death of a Child," *Journal for the Scientific Study of Religion* 22, no. 3 (1983): 222–38.

9. D. E. Balk. "Sibling Death, Adolescent Bereavement and Religion," *Death Studies* 15 (1991): 1–20.

10. H. G. Koenig, K. I. Pargament, and J. Nielsen. "Religious Coping and Health Status in Medically Ill Hospitalized Older Adults," *Journal of Nervous and Mental Disorders* 186 (1998): 513–21.

11. J. C. Hays, L. R. Landerman, L. K. George, E. P. Flint, H. G. Koenig, K. C. Land, and D. G. Blazer. "Social Correlates of the Dimensions of Depression in the Elderly," *Journal of Gerontology* (psychological sciences) 53B (1998): 31–9. Also: N. Krause, R. A. Herzog, and E. Baker. "Providing Support to Others and Well-Being in Later Life," *Journal of Gerontology* 47 (1992): 300–11.

12. This story was first reported in H. G. Koenig, T. Lamar, and B. Lamar, *A Gospel for the Mature Years: Finding Fulfillment by Knowing and Using your Gift* (Binghamton, NY: The Hayworth Press, 1997).

13. H. G. Koenig, H. J. Cohen, D. G. Blazer, C. Pieper, K. G. Meador, F. Shelp, V. Goli, and R. DiPasquale. "Religious Coping and Depression Among Elderly, Hospitalized Medically Ill Men," *American Journal of Psychiatry* 149, no. 12 (December 1992): 1693–1700.

14. H. G. Koenig, L. K. George, and B. L. Peterson. "Religiosity and Remission from Depression in Medically Ill Older Patients," *American Journal of Psychiatry* 155 (1998): 536–42.

15. J. K. Kiecolt-Glaser, and R. Glaser. "Psychoneuroimmunology and Health Consequences: Data and Shared Mechanisms," *Psychosomatic Medicine* 57 (1995): 269–74.

16. L. C. Kaldjian, J. F. Jekel, and G. Friedland. "End-of-Life Decisions in HIV-Positive Patients: The Role of Spiritual Beliefs," *AIDS* 12, no. 1 (1998): 103–7.

17. M. Galanter and P. Buckley. "Evangelical Religion and Meditation: Psychotherapeutic Effects," *Journal of Nervous and Mental Disease* 166 (1978): 685–91.

Chapter Seven: Religious People Live Longer, Healthier Lives

1. William J. Strawbridge, et al. "Frequent Attendance at Religious Services and Mortality over 28 Years," *American Journal of Public Health* 87, no. 6 (June 1997): 957–61.

2. D. B. Larson and H. G. Koenig. "Does Religion Prolong Life? A Systematic Review of Religion and Mortality," unpublished manuscript.

3. J. S. House, C. Robbins, and H. L. Metzner. "The Association of Social Relationships and Activities with Mortality: Prospective Evidence from the Tecumseh Community Health Study," *American Journal of Epidemiology* 116 (1982): 123–40.

4. D. M. Zuckerman, S. V. Kasl, and A. M. Ostfeld. "Psychosocial Predictors of Mortality Among the Elderly Poor," *American Journal of Epidemiology* 119 (1984): 410–23.

5. J. W. Dwyer, L. L. Clarke, and M. K. Miller. "The Effect of Religious Concentration and Affiliation on County Cancer Mortality Rates," *Journal of Health and Social Behavior* 31 (1990): 185–202.

6. J. F. Fries. "Aging, Natural Death, and the Compression of Morbidity," *New England Journal of Medicine* 303 (1980): 180–85.

7. J. V. Anthony, R. B. Terry, H. B. Hubert, and J. F. Fries. "Aging, Health Risks, and Cumulative Disability," *New England Journal of Medicine* 338 (April 9, 1998): 15.

8. E. I. Idler and S. V. Kasl. "Religion Among Disabled and Nondisabled Persons II: Attendance at Religious Services as a Predictor of the Course of Disability," *Journal of Gerontology* 52B no. 6 (1997): S306–S16.

Chapter Eight: Religion May Protect People from Serious Cardiovascular Disease

1. American Heart Association. *1998 Heart and Stroke Statistical Update* (Dallas: American Heart Association, 1997).

2. D. B. Larson, H. G. Koenig, B. H. Kaplan, R. F. Greenberg, E. Logue, and H. A. Tyroler. "The Impact of Religion on Blood Pressure Status in Men," *Journal of Religion and Health* 28 (1989): 265–78.

3. H. G. Koenig, L. K. George, H. J. Cohen, J. C. Hays, D. G. Blazer, and D. B. Larson. "The Relationship Between Religious Activities and Blood Pressure in Older Adults," *International Journal of Psychiatry in Medicine* 28 (1998): 189–213.

4. H. G. Koenig, L. K. George, H. J. Cohen, J. C. Hays, D. G. Blazer, and D. B. Larson. "The Relationship Between Religious Activities and Cigarette Smoking in Older Adults," *Journal of Gerontology* (medical sciences) 53A (1998): M426–M434.

5. Thomas E. Oxman, et al. "Lack of Social Participation or Religious Strength and Comfort as Risk Factors for Death after Cardiac Surgery in the Elderly," *Psychosomatic Medicine* 57 (1995): 5–15.

6. Y. Friedlander, J. D. Kark, and Y. Stein. "Religious Orthodoxy and Myocardial Infarction in Jerusalem: A Case Control Study," *International Journal of Cardiology* 10 (1986): 33–41.

7. Y. Friedlander, J. D. Kark, and Y. Stein. "Religious Observance and Plasma Lipids and Lipoproteins Among 17-Year-Old Jewish Residents of Jerusalem," *Preventive Medicine* 1 (January 16, 1987): 70–9.

8. N. Frasure-Smith, F. Lesperance, and M. Talajic. "Depression Following Myocardial Infarction, Impact on 6-Month Survival," *Journal of the American Medical Association* 270, no. 15 (October 20, 1993): 1819–25.

9. A. H. Glassman and P. A. Shapiro. "Depression and the Course of Coronary Artery Disease," *American Journal of Psychiatry* 155, no. 1 (January 1998): 4–11.

*

Chapter Nine: Religious People May Have Stronger Immune Systems

1. H. G. Koenig, H. J. Cohen, L. K. George, J. C. Hays, D. B. Larson, and D. G. Blazer. "Attendance at Religious Services, Interleukin-6, and Other Biological Parameters of Immune Function in Older Adults," *International Journal of Psychiatry in Medicine* 27, no. 3 (1997): 233–50.

2. H. G. Koenig and A. Futterman. "Religion and Health Outcomes: A Review and Synthesis of the Literature," Background paper, published in proceedings of *Conference on Methodological Approaches to the Study of Religion, Aging, and Health,* sponsored by the National Institute on Aging, March 16–17, 1995.

3. C. B. Nemeroff, K. R. Krishnan, D. Reed, R. Leder, C. Beam, and N. Dunick. "Adrenal Gland Enlargement in Major Depression: A Computed Tomographic Study," *Archives of General Psychiatry* 49, no. 5 (May 1992): 384–87.

4. R. T. Rubin, J. J. Phillips, T. F. Sadow, and J. T. McCracken. "Adrenal Gland Volume in Major Depression: Increase During the Depressive Episode and Decrease with Successful Treatment," *Archives of General Psychiatry* 52, no. 3 (March 1995): 213–18.

5. J. Leserman, J. M. Petitto, D. O. Perkins, J. D. Folds, R. N. Golden, and D. L. Evans. "Severe Stress, Depressive Symptoms, and Changes in Lymphocyte Subsets in Human Immunodeficiency Virus–Infected Men," *Archives of General Psychiatry* 54 (1997): 279–85.

6. H. J. Cohen, C. F. Pieper, T. Harris, K. M. K. Rao, and M. S. Currie. "The Association of Plasma IL-6 Levels with Functional Disability in Community Dwelling Elderly," *Journal of Gerontology* (medical sciences) 52A (1997): M201–8.

7. A. Fife, P. J. Beasley, and D. L. Fertig. "Psychoneuroimmunology and Cancer: Historical Perspectives and Current Research," *Advances in Neuroimmunology* 6 (1996): 179–90.

8. B. L. Andersen, et al. "Stress and Immune Responses After Surgical Treatment for Regional Breast Cancer," *Journal of the National Cancer Institute* 90, no. 1 (January 7, 1998): 30–6.

9. D. Spiegel. "Effects of Psychosocial Support on Patients with Metastatic

Breast Cancer," *Journal of Psychosocial Oncology* 10, no. 2 (1992): 115.

10. H. G. Prigerson, et al. "Traumatic Grief as a Risk Factor for Mental and Physical Morbidity," *American Journal of Psychiatry* 154, no. 5 (1997): 616–23.

11. S. J. Schleifer, et al. "Suppression of Lymphocyte Stimulation Following Bereavement," *Journal of the American Medical Association* 250, no. 3 (July 15, 1983): 374–77.

12. R. W. Bartrop, et al. "Depressed Lymphocyte Function After Bereavement," *The Lancet* (April 16, 1977): 834–36.

13. H. King, F. B. Locke. "American White Protestant Clergy as a Low-Risk Population for Mortality Research," *Journal of the National Cancer Institute* 65 (1980): 1115–24.

14. Y. F. Zhou, M. B. Leon, M. A. Waclawiw, J. J. Popma, Z. X. Yu, and S. E. Epstein. "Association Between Prior Cytomegalovirus Infection and the Risk of Restenosis After Coronary Atherectomy," *New England Journal of Medicine* 1335, no. 9 (August 29, 1996): 624–30.

15. F. J. Nieto, et al. "Coronary Heart Disease/Atherosclerosis/Myocardial Infarction: Cohort Study of Cytomegalovirus Infection as a Risk Factor For Carotid Intimal-Medial Thickening, a Measure of Subclinical Atherosclerosis," *Circulation* 94, no. 5 (September 1, 1996): 922–27.

16. T. E. Woods, M. H. Antoni, G. H. Ironson, and D. W. King. "Religiosity Associated with Affective and Immune Status in Symptomatic HIV-Infected Gay Men," *Journal of Psychosomatic Research* 46, no. 2 (1999): 165–76.

Chapter Ten: Religious People Use Fewer Expensive Hospital Services

1. S. R. Kunkel and R. A. Applebaum, "Estimating the Prevalence of Long-term Disability for an Aging Society," *Journal of Gerontology* 47 (1992): S253–60.

2. W. J. Meerding, et al. "Health-Care Cost of Ageing," *The Lancet* (January 10, 1998): 140.

3. H. G. Koenig. "Use of Acute Hospital Services and Mortality Among

Religious and Non-Religious Copers with Medical Illness," *Journal of Religious Gerontology* 9, no. 3 (1995): 1–22.

4. H. G. Koenig and D. B. Larson, "Use of Hospital Services, Religious Attendance, and Religious Affiliation," *Southern Medical Journal* 91, no. 10 (1998): 925–32.

5. E. McSherry. "The Scientific Basis of Whole Person Medicine," *Journal of American Scientific Affiliation* 35, no. 4 (1983): 217–24.

6. E. McSherry, D. Kratz, and W. A. Nelson. "Pastoral Care Departments: More Necessary in the DRG Era?" *Health Care Management Review* 11, no. 1 (1986): 58.

7. E. McSherry. "Outpatient Care: The Modern Chaplains' New Impact in Healthcare Reform," *Journal of Healthcare Chaplaincy* (Winter 1994).

8. Project IIR 89-045: Chaplin Visit Effect on Hospital Resource Use: Elisabeth McSherry, M.D., M.P.H., and William Nelson, Ph.D., M. Div. Brockton/West Roxbury VAMC, Brockton, MA; presented at VAMC research conference, Gainesville, FL, Feb. 7, 1997; full study under publishing review.

9. A. Trafford. "Can the Power of Prayer Be Measured?" *Washington Post*, Health, December 23, 1997: 6.

10. L. VandeCreek and B. Cooke. "Hospital Pastoral Care Practices of Parish Clergy," *Social Scientific Study of Religion* 7 (1996): 253–64.

Chapter Eleven: A Disease-Prevention Model for the Twenty-first Century

1. Department of Health and Human Services, Public Health Service, *Healthy People 2000, National Health Promotion and Disease Prevention* (Washington: DHHS Publication No. (PHS) 91-50212), p. 1.

2. J. S. Levin, D. B. Larson, and C. M. Puchalski. "Religion and Spirituality in Medicine: Research and Education," *Journal of the American Medical Association* 278, no. 9 (September 3, 1997): 792–93.

3. A. H. Glassman and P. A. Shapiro. "Depression and the Course of Coronary Artery Disease," *American Journal of Psychiatry* 155, no. 1 (January 1998): 4–11.

4. H. G. Koenig, et al. "Modeling the Cross-Sectional Relationships Between Religion, Physical Health, Social Support, and Depressive Symptoms," *American Journal of Geriatric Psychiatry* 5 (1997): 131–44.

5. J. K. Kieolt-Glaser and R. Glaser. "Psychoneuroimmunology and Health Consequences: Data and Shared Mechanisms," *Psychosomatic Medicine* 57 (1995): 269–70.

6. B. S. McEwen. "Protective and Damaging Effects of Stress Mediators," *New England Journal of Medicine* 383, no. 3 (January 15, 1998): 171–79.

7. A. H. Glassman and P. A. Shapiro. "Depression and the Course of Coronary Artery Disease," *American Journal of Psychiatry* 155, no. 1 (January 1998): 4–9.

8. R. C. Lefebvre, T. M. Lasater, R. A. Carleton, and G. Peterson. "Theory and Delivery of Health Programming in the Community: The Pawtucket Heart Health Program," *Preventive Medicine* 16, no. 1 (January 1987): 80–95. And: T. M. Lasater, B. L. Wells, R. A. Carleton, J. P. Elder. "The Role of Churches in Disease Prevention Research Studies," *Public Health Reports* 101, no. 2 (March–April 1986): 125–31.

9. "Patient Education & Counseling," *Patient Education Counseling* 19, no. 1 (February 1992): 19–32.

10. H. G. Koenig, L. K. George, K. G. Meador, D. G. Blazer, and S. M. Ford. "Religious Practices and Alcoholism in a Southern Adult Population," *Hospital & Community Psychiatry* 45 (1994): 225–37. And: K. A. Khavari and T. M. Harmon. "The Relationship Between Degree of Professed Religious Belief and Use of Drugs," *International Journal of Addictions* 17 (1982): 847–57.

11. K. S. Kendler, C. O. Gardner, and C. A. Prescott. "Religion, Psychopathology, and Substance Use and Abuse: A Multimeasure, Genetic-Epidemiologic Study," *American Journal of Psychiatry* 154, no. 3 (March 1997): 322.

12. J. W. Gardner and J. L. Lyon. "Low Incidence of Cervical Cancer in Utah," *Gynecologic Oncology* 5 (1977): 68–80.

13. L. J. Luecken, E. C. Suarez, C. M. Kuhn, J. C. Barefoot, J. A. Blumenthal, I. C. Siegler, and R. B. Williams. "Stress in Employed Women: Impact of Marital Status and Children at Home on Neurohormone Output and Home Strain," *Psychosomatic Medicine* 59, no. 4 (1997): 352–59.

Chapter Twelve: Helping Yourself and Your Loved Ones Benefit from the Power of Faith

1. K. Pargament, *The Psychology of Religion and Coping* (New York: The Guildford Press, 1997). And: H. G. Koenig, K. I. Pargament, and J. Nielsen, "Religious Coping and Health Status in Medically Ill Hospitalized Older Adults," 1998 *Journal of Nervous and Mental Disorders* 186, no. 9: 513–21.

❊
Suggested Further Reading

R. B. Byrd. "Positive Therapeutic Effects of Intercessory Prayer in a Coronary Care Unit Population," *Southern Medical Journal* 81 (1988): 826–29.

Bernard H. Fox. "The Role of Psychological Factors in Cancer Incidence and Prognosis," *Oncology* (March 1995): 245–53.

R. D. Hays, A. W. Stacy, K. F. Widaman, M. R. DiMatteo, and R. Downey. "Multistage Path Models of Adolescent Alcohol and Drug Use: A Reanalysis," *Journal of Drug Issues* 16, no. 3 (1986): 357–69.

G. Kennedy, W. Wisniewski, H. Kelman, C. Thomas, and H. Metz. "Religious Preference, Attendance at Services and the Prevalence of Depressive Symptoms in the Elderly," *Journal of Gerontology* 51B (December 1996): 301–8.

H. G. Koenig. *Aging and God* (Binghamton, NY: Haworth Press, 1994).

———. *A Gospel for the Mature Years* (Binghamton, NY: Haworth Press, 1997).

——— (ed.). *Handbook of Religion and Mental Health* (San Diego: Academic Press, 1998).

———. *Is Religion Good for Your Health?* (Binghamton, NY: Haworth Press, 1997).

H. G. Koenig, H. J. Cohen, D. G. Blazer, H. S. Kudler, K. R. R. Krishan, and T. E. Sibert. "Cognitive Symptoms of Depression and Religion Coping in Elderly Medical Patients," *Psychosomatics* 36 (1995): 369–75.

H. G. Koenig, I. C. Siegler, K. G. Meador, and L. K. George. "Religious Coping and Personality in Later Life," *International Journal of Geriatric Psychiatry* (1990): 5123–131.

G. Mathe. "Depression, Stressful Events and the Risk of Cancer," *Biomed & Pharmacother* 50 (1996): 1–2.

T. L. Saudia, M. R. Kinnery, K. C. Brown, and L. Young-Ward. "Health Locus of Control and Helpfulness of Prayer," *Heart and Lung* 20 (1991): 60–5.

F. K. Willits and D. M. Crider. "Religion and Well-Being: Men and Women in the Middle Years," *Review of Religious Research* 29, no. 3 (1988): 281–94.

✳ Index

*